CONTENTS

KU-484-841

WHO STUDY GROUP ON DIET, NUTRITION AND PREVENTION OF NONCOMMUNICABLE DISEASES

Geneva, 6–13 March 1989

*Members**

Professor G. Beaton, Department of Nutritional Sciences, University of Toronto, Canada

Dr Chen Chung-Ming, President, Chinese Academy of Preventive Medicine, Beijing, China (*Vice-Chairman*)

Dr A. Ferro-Luzzi, Director, Unit of Human Nutrition, National Institute of Nutrition, Rome, Italy

Professor M.K. Gabr,[†] Professor of Paediatrics, University of Cairo, Cairo, Egypt

Professor W.P.T. James, Director, The Rowett Research Institute, Aberdeen, Scotland (*Chairman*)

Dr K.A.V.R. Krishnamachari, Officer-in-Charge, Desert Medicine Research Centre, Jodhpur, India

Professor A.J. McMichael, Department of Community Medicine, University of Adelaide, Adelaide, Australia (*Rapporteur*)

Professor A. Omololu, University of Ibadan, Ibadan, Nigeria

Dr S. Palmer, Director, Food and Nutrition Board, National Academy of Sciences, Washington, DC, USA

Professor T.S. Sharmanov, Director, Institute of Regional Problems of Nutrition, Alma-Ata, USSR

Dr R. Suzue, Director, National Institute of Nutrition, Tokyo, Japan

Representatives of other organizations

Council for International Organizations of Medical Sciences
Dr Z. Bankowski
Food and Agriculture Organization of the United Nations
Dr K. Ge
International Council of Nurses
Miss K. McInerney
International Dental Federation
Professor D. Bratthall
International Diabetes Federation
Professor J.J. Hoet
International Life Sciences Institute
Professor R. Buzina

---

* Unable to attend: Dr A.M. O'Donnell, Centre for Studies on Infant Nutrition (CESNI), Buenos Aires, Argentina; Professor J. Stamler, Department of Community Health and Preventive Medicine, Northwestern University, Chicago, IL, USA (also representing the International Society and Federation of Cardiology).

[†] Also representing the International Union of Nutritional Sciences.

International Society of Dietetic Including All Infant and Young Children Food Industries
Dr J. Stanley
International Union against Cancer
Dr C. Mettlin
World Hypertension League
Dr T. Strasser

*Secretariat**

Dr E. Chigan, Director, Division of Noncommunicable Diseases, WHO, Geneva, Switzerland

Dr G. DeBacker, Department of Hygiene and Social Medicine, University Hospital, Ghent, Belgium (*Temporary Adviser*)

Dr I. Gyárfás, Chief, Cardiovascular Diseases, WHO, Geneva, Switzerland (*Co-secretary*)

Dr N.G. Khaltaev, Medical Officer, Division of Noncommunicable Diseases, WHO, Geneva, Switzerland

Professor D. Kromhout, Department of Epidemiology, National Institute of Public Health and Environmental Protection, Bilthoven, Netherlands (*Temporary Adviser*)

Dr R. MacLennan, Queensland Institute of Medical Research, Brisbane, Australia (*Temporary Adviser*)

Dr A.B. Miller, University of Toronto, Toronto, Canada (*Temporary Adviser*)

Professor G.P.M. Mwaluko, University of Dar-es-Salaam, Dar-es-Salaam, United Republic of Tanzania (*Temporary Adviser*)

Professor A. Nissinen, University of Kuopio, Kuopio, Finland (*Temporary Adviser*)

Dr A. Pradilla, Chief, Nutrition, WHO, Geneva, Switzerland

Dr K. Stanley, Cancer, WHO, Geneva, Switzerland (*Co-secretary*)

Dr J. Stjernswärd, Chief, Cancer, WHO, Geneva, Switzerland

Dr B. Torun, Institute of Nutrition of Central America and Panama (INCAP), Guatemala City, Guatemala (*Temporary Adviser*)

---

* Unable to attend: Dr P. Pietinen, Department of Epidemiology, National Public Health Institute, Helsinki, Finland (*Temporary Adviser*).

7

DIET, NUTRITION, AND THE PREVENTION OF CHRONIC DISEASES

Report of a WHO Study Group on Diet, Nutrition and Prevention of Noncommunicable Diseases

A WHO Study Group on Diet, Nutrition and Prevention of Noncommunicable Diseases met in Geneva from 6 to 13 March 1989. The meeting was opened by Dr Hu Ching-Li, on behalf of the Director-General, Dr Hiroshi Nakajima. He said that the amount and type of food eaten were fundamental determinants of human health. Since health was a fundamental determinant of the quality of each individual's life, good health should be a primary social goal. Improvements in the collective good health of a population—particularly the avoidance of chronic diseases in adult life—also decreased the costs associated with both health care and lost economic productivity. Good health was therefore an important economic asset.

Changes in dietary habits towards the "affluent" diet that prevailed in many developed countries had been followed by increases in the incidence of various chronic diseases of middle and later adult life. Initially, those chronic diseases coexisted with the long-standing and persistent problems associated with nutritional deficiencies, which could affect all age groups. The continuing public health importance of such deficiency disorders was recognized. However, the task of the Study Group was to provide recommendations that would help to prevent the chronic diseases that were related to the newly emerging dietary changes in developing countries, and to help in reducing the impact of these diseases in developed countries.

The Study Group's report would describe recent changes in the dietary and health patterns of countries, define the relationship between the "affluent" diet that typically accompanied economic development and the subsequent emergence of chronic diseases, and explore the need for national food and nutrition policies to prevent or minimize costly health problems in both developing and developed countries.

1. INTRODUCTION

1.1 Background

Over the course of evolution, human beings (and their primate predecessors) adapted progressively to a wide range of naturally occurring foods, but the types of food and the mix of nutrients (in terms of carbohydrates, fats, and protein) remained relatively constant throughout the ages. Food supply was often precarious, and starvation frequent.

The agricultural revolution, approximately 10 000 years ago, brought profound changes. The ability to produce and store food became more widespread, and some foods were preferentially cultivated. The industrial revolution in developed countries in the last 200 years has introduced radical changes in methods of food production, processing, storage, and distribution. Recent technological innovations, along with increased material well-being and life-styles that have allowed the exercise of dietary preferences (amplified by modern marketing techniques), have led to major changes in the nutritional composition of the diet in developed countries. For example, it is estimated that the per caput consumption of fat and sugar (refined carbohydrate) has increased 5–10-fold in England over the past 200 years, while the consumption of complex carbohydrates (including cereal grains) has declined substantially. Compared with the scale of human history and biological evolution, these developments represent dramatic and extremely rapid changes in population food supply.

The immediate health benefit of this increased and assured supply of food has been the elimination of starvation and the near-elimination of many micronutrient (e.g., vitamin) deficiency diseases in the developed countries of the world. The general improvement in nutritional status, with its associated increase in childhood growth rates, has brought an increased resistance to infectious disease. The overall effect has been to increase life expectancy substantially in many countries.

1.2 Diet-related chronic diseases: a recently identified problem

The longer-term adverse health effects of the "affluent" diet prevailing in the developed industrialized countries—characterized by an excess of energy-dense foods rich in fat and free sugars,[1] but a deficiency of complex carbohydrate foods (the main source of dietary fibre)—have only become apparent over recent decades. Epidemiological research has demonstrated a close and consistent relationship between the establishment of this type of diet and the emergence of a range of chronic non-infectious diseases— including, particularly, coronary heart disease, cerebrovascular disease, various cancers, diabetes mellitus, gallstones, dental caries, gastrointestinal disorders, and various bone and joint diseases.

Scientific evidence continues to accumulate supporting the important role of diet in the development of the most common causes of premature death in developed countries: cardiovascular diseases and cancer. Excess intake of saturated fats and elevated levels of blood cholesterol are linked with coronary heart disease —the most prevalent cardiovascular disease in the developed world. The main risk factor for stroke—the leading cardiovascular disorder in many developing countries—is high blood pressure, in which obesity, alcohol intake, and excess salt intake play major contributory roles. Obesity is also strongly related to the onset of diabetes. It has been estimated that approximately one-third of cancers are associated with dietary factors. For example, an excess intake of fat has been linked to an increased incidence of cancers of the breast and colon.

The dynamic relationship between changes in a population's diet and changes in its health has been well reflected in the rapidly changing disease and mortality profiles of migrant populations moving from low-risk to high-risk countries (e.g., from Japan to the USA). It has also been evident in some countries, e.g., China, Mauritius, Singapore, and those in the Caribbean, that have undergone rapid development over the past 40–50 years.

This population-based evidence of the importance of diet has been amplified and confirmed by recent epidemiological studies in which information has been obtained from large numbers of individuals. The identity of the specific components of diet that increase the probability of occurrence of these diseases in individuals is being clarified. For some dietary risk factors, particularly in relation to cardiovascular diseases, there is recent epidemiological

---

[1] For the purposes of this report, the Study Group considered the term "free sugars" to include monosaccharides, disaccharides, and other short-chain sugars produced by refining carbohydrates.

11

evidence that a reduced consumption can lower the incidence of disease.

The causes of these chronic diseases are complex, and dietary factors are only part of the explanation. Individuals also differ in their susceptibility to the adverse health effects of specific dietary factors, but within the public health context the focus is the health of whole populations. Public health interventions aim to lower the *average* level of risk to health of whole populations, either because the whole population is at risk, or because a strategy to identify the minority of individuals at greatest risk, even if available, would only contribute to a modest public health improvement, since much if not most of the disease in the population occurs in the more numerous individuals at moderate to low risk.

1.3 The population perspective

Within any one population, the medical care system can sometimes develop approaches to reducing the risk of disease in certain individuals, particularly those at high risk. Thus, physicians may give dietary advice in order to lower the blood cholesterol level in a high-risk individual who has a strong family history of coronary heart disease or a raised blood cholesterol level.

From the clinical viewpoint, the health risk status of an individual is typically assessed by comparison with equivalent health risk measurements made on other members of the population. Thus, an individual's blood pressure or blood cholesterol concentration might be deemed to be "high" if, for example, it exceeds the levels present in three-quarters of the population. That is, the individual's health risks are viewed relative to those of other individuals in that population.

But from the population perspective, it may be that the entire population's risk profile is "high" relative to other populations. Thus, the public health approach to disease prevention requires health-oriented nutrition and food policies for whole populations. This has also been referred to as "mass intervention". For example, in developed countries populations with high average levels of blood cholesterol warrant food and nutrition policies (i.e., public health policies) directed at displacing that population's distribution of blood cholesterol levels to a lower range. Populations in developing countries, with their lower average levels of blood cholesterol, should also adopt food and nutrition policies—but in their case the aim should be to avoid future increases in blood cholesterol levels.

This report is about primary prevention at the population level. In developing countries, the aim should be to avoid the diseases and premature deaths related to the "affluent" diet that characterizes the populations of many developed countries. In the developed countries, the aim should be to moderate or remove the excesses in the present diet that contribute to the high incidence of these diseases.

Developing countries can benefit by learning from the experience of dietary change and adverse health effects in many developed countries. If they act now, the governments of developing countries can gain for their people the health benefits of avoiding nutritional deficiencies without encouraging the development of the chronic diet-related diseases that usually accompany economic and technological development. Thus, as well as reduced childhood mortality, increased life expectancy should be sought by means of nutrition policies that minimize diet-related chronic disease, thereby avoiding the social and economic costs of premature death during the period of highest economic activity, in middle age. These nutritional policies will also improve the quality of life in the elderly.

1.4 Achieving population-based dietary change

If such a socially and economically desirable goal is to be achieved, then national governments in both developing and developed countries must:

1. Be aware of the relationship between the changes in a population's diet that tend to accompany economic development and the consequent changes in the health of the population.
2. Recognize that it is both possible and desirable to seek an optimum national diet, in association with economic development, that both maximizes health benefits and minimizes health hazards.
3. Develop nutrition-based health policies that are intersectoral. These should involve many government departments, and be supported by the activities of nongovernmental organizations, health care workers, and the community at large. Such widespread involvement is needed in order to influence favourably the production, processing, and marketing of foods conducive to health, and to increase public awareness of the

13

relationship between food and health. The mix of integrated policies will constitute a progressive, health-oriented, national food and nutrition policy. From the individual's point of view, such a policy will make healthy choices when purchasing food the easy choices.

Intersectoral public policies are difficult to develop. The links between diet, nutrition, and health have often been poorly specified, and it has therefore been difficult to bring the issues into focus as a coherent public policy. The priority traditionally given in national budgets to food production, without regard to the effects on the consumers' nutrition and health, needs to be reconsidered. Short-term policies that seek to maximize local economic activity and foreign exchange earnings, while neglecting health considerations, may incur substantial health care costs and loss of productivity in economically important groups of the community.

Economic development is normally accompanied by improvements in a country's food supply as regards both quantity and quality (i.e., less spoilage and less contamination of food). Provision of a nutritionally adequate and hygienic diet, in a socially equitable fashion, confers major health benefits, including:

- Elimination of dietary deficiency diseases.
- Reduction of acute and chronic foodborne diseases.
- Improvements in overall nutritional status, including increased childhood growth rates.
- Increased resistance to bacterial and parasitic infectious diseases.

A major consequence of improvements in the food supply has been an increase in life expectancy. However, further economic development has entailed qualitative changes in the production, processing, distribution, and marketing of food. With these changes have come the problems of diet-related chronic diseases, which typically occur in middle and later adult life, and counteract the gains in life expectancy attributable to an improved food supply. These chronic diseases are, in part, manifestations of nutrient excesses and imbalances in the "affluent" diet, so they are in principle largely preventable.

In developed countries, the enormous cost of the high-technology, tertiary health care needed for the diagnosis and management of these high-incidence chronic diseases is already apparent. Similar demands in developing countries will impose a huge burden on the human and economic resources of the country and are liable to disturb priorities in the health care sector.

In many developed countries, there is now growing evidence of social and political acceptance of the need for prevention-oriented health policies and behaviour to reduce the incidence of diet-related chronic diseases. Some developed countries have been active in public education, using national dietary guidelines as a stimulus. Changes in consumer preferences (e.g., for foods lower in salt, free sugars, and saturated fat, but higher in dietary fibre) have emerged, initially in the upper socioeconomic groups. These changes in preference are leading to modification of systems for food production and processing. Progress in changing consumer preferences is intrinsically slow, and so far has occurred largely without any support from public policies in any but the health sectors.

Despite this limited support, mortality from coronary heart disease (the leading cause of death in developed countries) has begun to decline and there has been a reduction in the prevalence of hypertension in many developed countries. The downturns have been particularly strong—with, for example, a fall of 40–50% in deaths due to coronary heart disease over the past 20 years in North America and Australia. These recent reductions in death rate reflect changes in population life-style, e.g., in dietary habits, such as decreases in the consumption of saturated fats.

The process of changing unsatisfactory dietary practices and promoting health in developed countries can prove socially and politically difficult. Similarly, there will be difficulties in developing countries, even if action is needed to avoid dangerous trends rather than to reverse them. Inappropriate public perceptions in developing countries of what constitutes a better diet, and the economic pressures to establish local food industries based on products with high contents of fat, sugar, and salt, are already evident. These issues must be confronted and dealt with if the suffering and economic impact of cardiovascular diseases, cancers, and other diet-related chronic diseases are to be avoided.

In some developing countries, the first priority must remain the attainment of an adequate food supply for the whole population and the elimination of various forms of nutritional deficiency among vulnerable groups (e.g., protein–energy, vitamin, and mineral deficiencies). However, as in the developed countries, efforts are also required to forestall or arrest a population shift towards a high intake of saturated fat, sugar, and salt. This shift is now occurring almost everywhere, even if only in some sectors of society. The challenge is therefore to know how best to formulate health-oriented national policies for food that can provide the usual health gains associated with economic development while minimizing the future social and economic costs of the diet-related chronic diseases of adult life that will emerge if developing countries follow the previous experience of many countries in the developed world.

2. CHANGES IN PATTERNS OF DISEASE IN RELATION TO CHANGES IN DIET

This section summarizes the long-standing health problems caused by nutritional deficiencies. It then explores the widespread emergence of the more "affluent" type of diet that has accompanied economic development and urbanization and is associated with an increase in the incidence of many chronic diet-related diseases of adult life.

2.1 Deficiency diseases

2.1.1 *Protein–energy malnutrition*

Undernutrition, malnutrition, and the widespread prevalence of communicable diseases have been the major health and welfare problems facing developing countries for the last 50 years. After the Second World War, medical research revealed a host of nutritional disorders in many developing countries, e.g., pellagra, and vitamin A- and iodine-deficiency states. Protein–energy malnutrition was recognized as a widespread and important public health problem in all regions of the developing world. Methods of defining protein–energy malnutrition in children and adults were developed for use in both a clinical and a public health context. The growth of children and the size of adults reflect the effects of diet, infection, psychosocial and genetic factors, and, indirectly, agricultural and economic influences. Anthropometric measures are therefore one index of the nutritional state of the individual or community.

More recently, it has become clear that the resistance of children and adults to infectious diseases often depends on their nutritional state, which can have a profound impact on the development of immunity. Given this perspective, and the rapidly expanding populations of many developing countries, economic planning for the health services and for agriculture has properly emphasized the importance of a clean water supply and environmental improvements to reduce waterborne parasitic and enteric infections; childhood immunization programmes; a hygienic and nutritionally adequate diet to prevent malnutrition, deficiency diseases, foodborne infections, and intoxication; and the equitable distribution of resources within the population.

Once water quality and food sufficiency and safety have been addressed at national level, economic planning comes to be dominated by considerations other than health issues. Hence, many governments now emphasize the importance of improving the economic welfare of subsistence farmers who, in a number of developing countries, constitute the majority of the population. Import/export policies, agrarian reform, food subsidies, rural development schemes, and, more recently, economic structural adjustments usually dominate the making of economic and agricultural policies at both national and international levels.

Over the last 20 years, substantial progress has been made in making food available (Table 1) and in improving health, although the sub-Saharan region of Africa remains of extreme concern in relation to food supplies (Table 2). In Africa, there is a clear concordance between the FAO estimates of national food availability in 1979–1981 (Table 2) and the prevalence of underweight children in each country. More recently collated anthropometric data for children in different African countries confirm these relationships.

The extremely difficult economic, agricultural, and health circumstances of sub-Saharan Africa should not obscure the dramatic changes in the health status of many of the urban communities in the region, and the major advances in agriculture and health care made in the rest of the world. In these other regions there has been, despite a huge increase in population, a rise in per caput food production. Indices of general nutritional status, as well as of health care, have also shown substantial improvements, with progressive declines in the proportion of low-birth-weight babies and of wasted children, and in infant and child mortality.

Over the last 25 years, China's food production has increased substantially and its population by about 60%; dietary energy supply increased from less than 1800 $kcal_{th}$ (7.53 MJ) per caput per

Table 1. Trends in per caput dietary energy supplies, by region and economic group [a]

Region	Period A 1961–63 (kcal$_{th}$ per caput per day)	Period B 1981–83 (kcal$_{th}$ per caput per day)	% increase A–B
Developed countries	3110	3390	9
Developing countries	1980	2400	21
Developing market economies	2060	2340	14
—Africa	2120	2230	5
—"Far East" [b]	1940	2190	13
—Latin America	2370	2620	11
—"Near East" [b]	2230	2900	30
Asian centrally planned economies	1830	2540	39
World	2340	2660	14

[a] Adapted from reference 1, by kind permission of the Food and Agriculture Organization of the United Nations.
[b] As defined by FAO, see reference 1.

Table 2. Daily per caput dietary energy supplies for the 20 most populous countries in Africa south of the Sahara, 1979–81 [a]

< 2000 kcal$_{th}$	Burkina Faso
	Ghana
	Mali
	Mozambique
	Uganda
2001–2300 kcal$_{th}$	Cameroon
	Ethiopia
	Kenya
	Malawi
	Zaire
	Zambia
	Zimbabwe
> 2300 kcal$_{th}$	Angola
	Côte d'Ivoire
	Madagascar
	Nigeria
	Senegal
	South Africa
	Sudan
	United Republic of Tanzania

[a] Adapted from reference 1, by kind permission of the Food and Agriculture Organization of the United Nations.

day in 1961–63 to 2560 kcal$_{th}$ (10.71 MJ) in 1983–85. There were corresponding increases in birth weights and childhood growth rates, and infant mortality fell from 200 (per 1000 live births) before 1949 to about 40 in 1980, and to 35 in 1982. Improvements in sanitation, health care, the control of communicable diseases, and diet account for this reduction in mortality.

In many regions, e.g., southern Asia, South America, and northern Africa, infant mortality is still high, but in most countries it continues to decline. Trends in anthropometric data for children under five years of age indicate that the prevalence of wasting (i.e., the proportion of children less than two standard deviations below the reference weight-for-height) and of low birth weight (the proportion of infants weighing less than 2500 g at birth) has decreased significantly in the last two decades. In the WHO regions of the Americas, Eastern Mediterranean, Europe, and Western Pacific, many national averages for wasting and low birth weight are below 8%. In parts of southern Asia and Africa, wasting is still a major public health problem, and national averages also hide the existence of differences and inequalities among various socio-economic groups within the same country.

Growth failure (stunting) remains widespread in most of the developing world. Although the overall trends indicate an improvement in growth, the average rates of growth in childhood may be decreasing in some African countries. The decrease in the proportion of wasted and stunted children has unfortunately been outweighed by large increases in the total populations of South-East Asia and Africa, so that the net result has been an increase in the total number of wasted and stunted children in Africa, and no change in Asia.

While acute childhood malnutrition is, in general, a receding problem, large populations of children and adults, especially in Africa, are nevertheless subsisting on inadequate food supplies in times of drought.

There is also widespread chronic undernutrition around the world, causing growth retardation among children and affecting physical and psychosocial development, as described later (section 4.1.1). Continuous surveillance and appropriate interventions are needed in many countries, particularly in areas affected by natural and man-made crises and by economic recession.

Many epidemiological studies have linked a low intake of animal protein to high childhood mortality, morbidity, and growth failure. For many years, this evidence was interpreted as meaning that the amino acids present in animal protein were necessary to complement the amino acids in plant foods. (Most animal sources contain the complete range of essential amino acids, while many plant sources are low in one or more.) Progressively it was recognized that, even in totally vegetarian diets containing a diversity of foods, plant sources tended to complement one another in amino acid supply. Although the total amount of protein in the diet may need to be higher in vegetarian diets to provide an adequate intake of all the amino acids, the usual concentrations of proteins in these diets are sufficient. If the energy needs of the child or adult are met by these diets—then so are the amino acid needs. With this evolution of understanding, a reconsideration of the epidemiological data suggested that the apparent "animal protein effect" on childhood growth and health was not necessarily a biological effect related to protein supply as such. Animal protein consumption might instead be serving as an index of more affluent household conditions that affected both buying power and living conditions. Alternatively, animal food sources may be improving health by counteracting micronutrient deficiencies. There is strong evidence that, as income constraints are relieved in most developing societies, there is a spontaneous demand for increased intakes of foods of animal origin. Studies continue to show a positive association between intake of such foods and a range of improved functions (physical and psychological) among the deprived segments of many populations. However, it has not been shown scientifically that increasing the consumption of such foods will, in itself, improve these human functions.

It should be recognized that, at some stages of life, there continue to be strong nutritional reasons for advocating at least modest intakes of foods of animal origin. Even more importantly, the risk of deficiencies of protein and other nutrients may increase as the range of different foods in individual diets becomes more limited. Diversity in the availability and use of foods must therefore continue to be a key component of any programme aimed at maintaining, or improving, the nutritional health of the population. A policy to limit the consumption of saturated fatty acids should not be simplified to signify a need to limit foods of animal origin whatever their fat content.

In agrarian societies it is now clear that consideration must be given not only to the supply of food and nutrients but also to the short- and long-term effects of agricultural policies upon the income and buying power of the small producers. In turn, as urban migration proceeds, policies must be adjusted to take account of the differential impact on an urban cash economy and on a rural subsistence economy of agricultural and dietary changes. There is a need to strive for equity in both population groups, while ensuring a nutritionally adequate and appropriate diet.

2.1.2 *Iodine deficiency disorders*

Iodine deficiency disorders are a major scourge and their prevention or amelioration depends on the ready availability of iodine in the water consumed by the population, or in the types of food eaten. The Andes, Alps, Great Lakes basin of North America, and the Himalayas are particularly iodine-deficient mountainous areas, but coastal areas and plains may also be deficient. Excessive intakes of goitrogens (for example from consumption of cassava in central Africa, or of waterborne goitrogens in Latin America) interfere with the normal uptake and metabolism of iodine and can thus amplify the effects of iodine deficiency.

In addition to the clinically obvious and easily recognizable effects of iodine deficiency (i.e., goitre and cretinism), the more pervasive effects of milder iodine deficiency on the survival and physical and mental development of children, intellectual ability, and the work capacity of adults are now being recognized. Iodine deficiency disorders (2) are of sufficient importance to warrant urgent government action and monitoring, since about one thousand million people are affected in more than 80 countries.

Elsewhere in this report, recommendations are made that if adopted would lead, for many countries, to reduced salt consumption. Iodination of salt is one of the very few effective ways of controlling endemic goitre, and indeed there is some indication that the problem is increasing in some sections of Europe as people voluntarily reduce salt usage. In areas where iodine intakes from other sources are low, there is a clear need for coordination of policies relating to the control of goitre by iodination of salt and to the control of hypertension risk by limiting salt intake. There may be a need to adjust the iodination levels of salt as salt intake changes or, in industrialized countries, to add iodine to all salt rather than only to table salt.

2.1.3 *Vitamin A deficiency*

Vitamin A deficiency, leading to xerophthalmia and sometimes blindness, continues to be a widespread problem among children (Fig. 1). Deficiency of vitamin A also decreases resistance to

21

Fig. 1. The geographical distribution of xerophthalmia in 1987 [a]

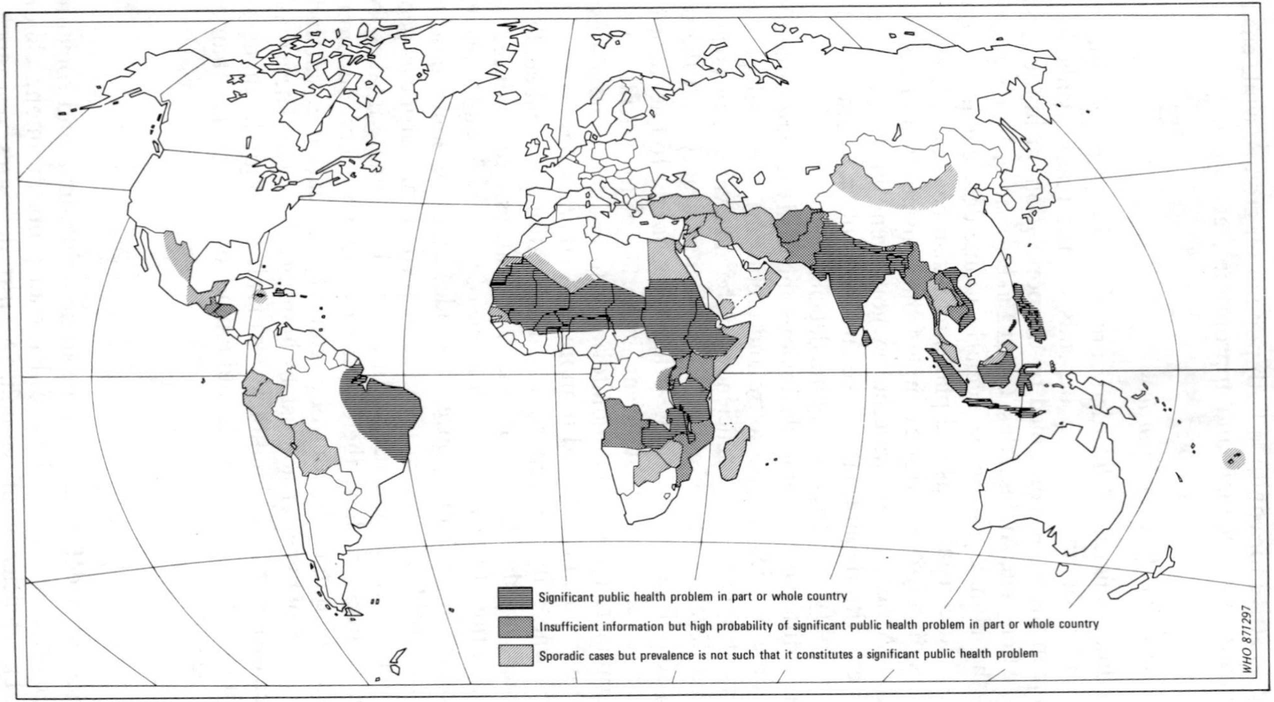

WHO 871297

Significant public health problem in part or whole country

Insufficient information but high probability of significant public health problem in part or whole country

Sporadic cases but prevalence is not such that it constitutes a significant public health problem

[a] Adapted and updated from reference 3, by kind permission of the International Pediatric Association.

infections and increases mortality. There is now some evidence that vitamin A supplements in deficient populations can reduce both mortality and blindness. Analyses of food supplies from different regions show that the availability of vitamin A is limited; this problem is exacerbated by any tendency to withhold vegetables from children for cultural or other reasons. In Asia, there is a particular problem because the estimated overall average availability of vitamin A is less than that required by the population. Any maldistribution of foods high in vitamin A within the population would further exacerbate the problem. Although in most countries there is a slow but steady improvement in the availability of foods rich in vitamin A (Fig. 2), xerophthalmia continues to be a major problem in about 40 countries.

Elsewhere in this report, emphasis is placed upon the desirability of low-fat diets for the prevention of cardiovascular disease and cancer. Very low fat intakes will interfere with the absorption of vitamin A and provitamin A. However, at the levels of fat advocated in this report, i.e., 15–30% of energy, no detrimental effects on absorption would be expected.

2.1.4 Iron deficiency

A further example of a continuing deficiency disease of wide-spread importance is anaemia. Table 3 shows the startling difference in the prevalence of anaemia at all ages in developing compared with developed countries. Africa and southern Asia have a particular problem, the dominant cause being iron deficiency. Intestinal parasitosis exacerbates iron deficiency by increasing the loss of blood from the intestine. This loss, in association with a low intake of iron and/or its poor absorption, can lead to profound anaemia, which impairs the intellectual development of children and limits both children's and adults' capacity for physical activity. In Africa, Asia, and South America, the trend in iron availability has been deteriorating rather than improving (Fig. 2), so it is not surprising that iron deficiency anaemia continues to be a massive public health problem in the world. There is also some evidence of anaemia occurring among young children, pregnant women, and the elderly in industrialized countries.

The availability of dietary iron for absorption is affected by both the form of iron and the nature of the foods concurrently ingested. Two major forms of iron exist in diets—haem iron and "inorganic"

Fig. 2. Changes in availability of vitamin A, iron, and energy, by FAO region, from 1960/65 to 1975/77 [a]

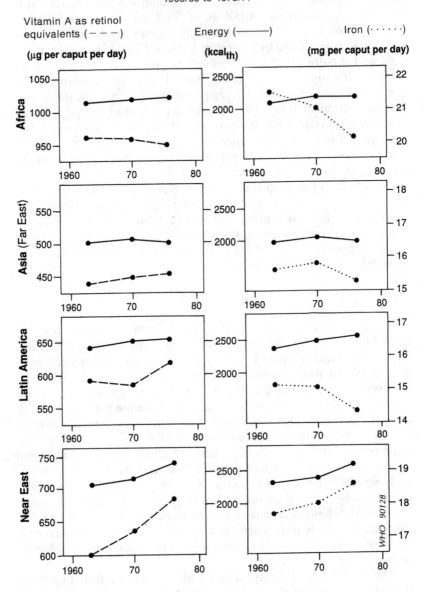

[a] Reproduced with permission from reference 4. Far East and Near East as defined by FAO, see reference 1.

24

Table 3. Estimated prevalence of anaemia and number affected, by geographical region and age/sex category, around 1980 (population data in millions)[a, b]

Region	Children				Men 15–59 years		Women 15–49 years			
	0–4 years		5–12 years				Pregnant		All women	
	%	No.	%	No.	%	No.	%	No.	%	No.
Africa	56	48.0	49	47.3	20	23.4	63	11.3	44	46.8
North America	8	1.6	13	3.6	4	3.1	–	–	8	5.1
Latin America	26	13.7	26	18.1	13	12.8	30	3.0	17	14.7
Eastern Asia[c]	20	3.2	22	5.6	11	6.1	20	0.5	18	8.4
Southern Asia	56	118.7	50	139.2	32	123.6	65	27.1	58	191.0
Europe	14	4.7	5	2.7	2	3.0	14	0.8	12	14.1
Oceania	18	0.4	15	0.5	7	0.5	25	0.1	19	1.0
Developed regions	12	10.3	7	9.1	3	12.0	14	2.0	11	32.7
Developing regions	51	183.2	46	208.3	26	162.2	59	41.9	47	255.7
World	43	193.5	37	217.4	18	174.2	51	43.9	35	288.4

[a] Adapted from reference 5.
[b] Anaemia is defined as a haemoglobin concentration below WHO reference values for age, sex, and pregnancy status (see WHO Technical Report Series, No. 405, 1968).
[c] Excluding China.

iron. The former, found only in animal sources, is readily available and absorption is not influenced by other constituents of the diet. Absorption of inorganic iron is strongly influenced by factors present in foods ingested at the same time. Two widely recognized promoters of absorption are animal foods and ascorbic acid (vitamin C). Even though diets based primarily on cereals and legumes may contain much iron, without coexistent factors such as vitamin C, they may actually provide only a low level of available iron (6).

Concern about iron deficiency is one nutritional reason for recommending the consumption of at least some meat, or foods providing a substantial amount of ascorbic acid.

2.1.5 Fluoride deficiency

There is clear clinical, epidemiological, and experimental evidence that fluoride significantly reduces the incidence of dental caries (7). Until about 10 years ago it was believed that fluorides worked principally by increasing the resistance of enamel to acids produced in dental plaque from sugars. More recent research clearly shows that fluoride acts principally by remineralizing the early carious lesion and by an effect on the bacteria in dental plaque. Fluoride intake may be increased to optimum levels by fluoridation of community water supplies, by adding fluoride to salt, milk, or toothpaste, by taking fluoride supplements, or by the topical application of fluoride.

The combined effect of fluoride sufficiency and a lowered intake of free sugars (including sucrose) is beneficial in terms of the development of caries (see section 3.8). The consumption of a limited amount of free sugars is acceptable only if the population is using fluoridated toothpaste and/or drinking fluoridated water.

2.1.6 Vitamin B_{12} deficiency

Vitamin B_{12} deficiency causes anaemia and, if severe, neurological disorders. It is of concern with vegetarian diets containing no animal foods. Vitamin B_{12} is a product of bacterial fermentation, such as occurs in the intestine of ruminant animals such as cattle, sheep, and goats. Meat and milk are major sources of vitamin B_{12}. Some may be contributed also by fermented foods. The need for vitamin B_{12} has therefore been a part of the rationale for recommending the consumption of animal foods. The levels of animal foods recommended in this report would be ample to supply the dietary needs for this vitamin (6).

Pernicious anaemia, a severe vitamin B_{12} deficiency secondary to a defect in the absorption of vitamin B_{12}, occurs with low incidence in all societies, and is unaffected by the dietary level of vitamin B_{12}, or the nature of the diet.

2.1.7 Other nutrient deficiencies and excesses

Only the major deficiencies have been mentioned above. Other significant disorders include:

1. Rickets, which is still widespread in parts of northern Africa and the eastern Mediterranean, and is reported to be increasing in Mexico; this condition is attributable to insufficient exposure to sunlight and lack of vitamin D in the diet.
2. Ascorbic acid deficiency, particularly in some drought-affected populations, e.g., in Africa.
3. Deficiencies of other trace elements, e.g., of zinc.

4. Excessive intakes of certain vitamins and minerals (e.g., vitamin A/carotene, vitamin D, selenium, and fluorine), which can occur as a result of prolonged or acute overdosage, usually in affluent countries. The subject of fluorosis is discussed elsewhere (section 3.8).

2.1.8 *Conclusion on the importance of deficiencies*

While in most parts of the world there have been significant advances in the control of protein–energy deficiency and specific nutritional disorders, in all regions of the world there are still some populations affected by one or more of these deficiencies. In some regions, the number of undernourished people is increasing even if the proportion is declining. Even the trends in prevalence are unfavourable in some countries. While the emphasis in this report is on preventing the diseases related to overnutrition or to excesses of certain elements in the diet, for the majority of countries there is still a need for vigorous policies and action to combat the various deficiency disorders, as part of comprehensive health-oriented national food and nutrition policies. Improvement is needed in the quality as well as the quantity of the diet, but greater quantities of food are particularly important in sub-Saharan Africa and southern Asia.

As a guide for policy-makers, recommended dietary intakes for energy, vitamins, and minerals to avoid deficiencies are given in Annex 1.

2.2 Emerging diet-related chronic diseases

While some developing countries remain concerned with the problems of hunger and malnutrition, and communicable diseases, in other countries there have been considerable increases in the prevalence of chronic diseases. For example, during the 1970s, mortality from these diseases underwent a relative increase of 105% in tropical South America and 56% in Central America, Mexico, and Panama (Table 4). Similar increases in these diseases are occurring in developing countries in all regions of the world.

Rapid changes are occurring in the life-styles and the dietary and health patterns of the populations in developing countries. There has been a huge increase in the numbers of people moving from rural to

Table 4. Changes in the percentage of total mortality due to chronic diseases in five subregions of the Americas between 1970 and 1980 [a]

Subregion	Percentage mortality attributed to chronic diseases (1980)	Relative % increase (1970–1980)
North America (USA and Canada)	75	0.4
Temperate South America (Southern Cone countries)	60	11
Caribbean area	57	21
Tropical South America	45	105
Continental Middle America (Central America, Mexico and Panama)	28	56

[a] Adapted from reference 8.

urban communities, where striking changes in diet often occur (see section 2.2.1).

Table 5 shows that obesity in adults is not confined to the industrialized countries. Obesity is already prevalent in the developing world, particularly in women, with very high rates in some places, e.g., in Trinidad. The prevalence of obesity is surprisingly variable, but in some developing countries high rates are already evident in children as well as in adults (Fig. 3). As life expectancy increases in many developing countries, new problems of cardiovascular disorders and cancers are emerging; these reflect the coexisting effects of the demographic "aging" of the population and of newly acquired risks relating to the diets and life-styles that have accompanied economic development. On current trends, such diseases will present a huge health-care burden for less affluent communities in the near future.

The stage at which cardiovascular disease emerges as a significant cause of death corresponds to a life-expectancy level between 50 and 60 years, and at this level cardiovascular disease mortality accounts for 15–25% of all deaths. This analysis reflects cross-sectional data from different countries, but the pattern has been confirmed by longitudinal studies of the evolving pattern of disease and life expectancy in many developed as well as developing societies. Cardiovascular diseases were on average already becoming a significant cause of death in developing countries between 1970 and 1975, whereas the corresponding period in the USA was about 50 years earlier, i.e., in the 1920s. On current projections, cardiovascular diseases will emerge or be established as a substantial health problem in virtually every country in the world by the year 2000.

Table 5. Prevalence of obesity in adults in national surveys as indicated by a body-mass index (BMI) greater than 30[a, b]

Country or area	Age group (years)	Percentage obese	
		Male	Female
Costa Rica	40–45	5.7	14.4
El Salvador	40–45	0.0	1.5
Guatemala	40–45	0.0	5.6
Honduras	40–45	2.8	6.0
Nicaragua	40–45	3.1	16.4
Panama	40–45	2.3	1.7
Trinidad (urban)	40	–	32.0
Australia	35–44	6.2	7.5
Canada	–	8.5	9.3
Netherlands	35–49	4.2	5.0
United Kingdom	35–49	7.9	8.6
United States of America	–	12.0	15.0

[a] Adapted from reference 9.
[b] BMI = body mass in kg/(height in metres)^2.

Good data from Africa are limited, but Mauritius has experienced a 65% increase in death rates from both coronary heart disease and breast cancer over the last 30 years. These diseases are already becoming a burden on hospitals in the capitals of the sub-Saharan countries, where they particularly affect the middle classes. These affluent groups have already changed their diets from the traditional foods and increased their smoking. In several Asian, Caribbean, and Latin American countries, the problem of breast cancer is evident, and although there is variation from country to country, the emergence of coronary heart disease is also apparent. In some countries, divergent trends have occurred. For example, in Japan, the incidence of breast cancer is increasing as diets change, but the reduction in hypertension seems to have overridden the effect of an increasing intake of saturated fat, such that Japanese national rates for coronary heart disease have been falling.

Population surveys carried out since 1970 in developing countries show that the prevalence of hypertension ranges from 1% to 30% in some African countries to over 30% in Brazil (10, 11). In many Latin American countries, death rates from hypertensive disease and stroke are declining, changes also ascribed to the effects of dietary alterations. The prevalence of hypertension is low in rural areas of developing countries, where the diet is low in salt.

Table 6 shows the estimated life expectancy of individuals in countries from the different regions in the 1950s and 1980s, and the changes projected for the years 2020–2025. Every region of the world

Fig. 3. Prevalence of obesity in preschool children, defined as a weight more than two standard deviations above the reference median weight-for-height[a, b]

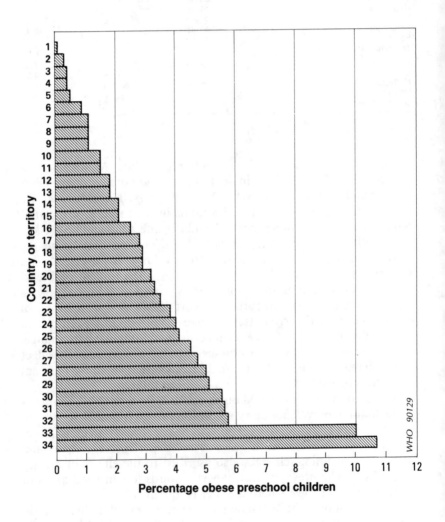

Country or area	Notes[c]
1. Papua New Guinea	Kar Kar, Lufa
2. Bangladesh	Rural
3. Philippines	
4. Burkina Faso	Mossi Tribe
5. Singapore	
6. Togo	Gourma Tribe
7. Tunisia	1–4.99 years
8. Rwanda	
9. India	Kerala
10. Indonesia	East Java
11. Belize	
12. Jordan	Amman (rural)
13. Tahiti	
14. Nicaragua	
15. Brazil	Paraiba
16. Saint Lucia	
17. United Kingdom	
18. Yugoslavia	Zagorje (rural)
19. Antigua	
20. Zambia	
21. Venezuela	
22. Italy	1–4.99 years
23. Panama	
24. Peru	
25. Barbados	
26. Honduras	Suyapa, 0–2.99 years
27. Lesotho	
28. Bolivia	Montero Region
29. Trinidad and Tobago	
30. Iran (Islamic Republic of)	Rural
31. Mauritius	
32. Canada	
33. Jamaica	
34. Chile	0–5.99 years

[a] Reproduced from reference 9.
[b] Reference population of the National Center for Health Statistics, USA.
[c] Children aged 0–59 months unless otherwise stated.

has seen an increase in life expectancy over the last 30 years, and this is expected to increase markedly in Africa and Asia over the next 30 years.

As infant and childhood mortality declines, the proportion, and total numbers, of people living into old age can be expected to increase rapidly. Table 7 shows the projected increase in the numbers of elderly, aged 60 years and over, by the year 2025. A substantial increase in numbers is expected even in Africa and Asia, where the expected age structure will still be dominated by children and young adults. Asia and Latin America will have a proportion of elderly in 2025 that exceeds the proportion observed in the more affluent communities in the 1950s.

Thus, it can be predicted that in all regions of the world there will be many millions of older adults who, although immune to many infections, will be susceptible to cardiovascular diseases and cancers. Table 8 shows the causes of death in the developed and developing world in 1980. Clearly, infectious and parasitic diseases are still of immense significance in the developing world, but cardiovascular diseases and cancer already account for over a fifth of all deaths. If deaths in infancy and childhood are excluded, then these chronic diseases assume much greater significance.

Table 6. Trends in life expectancy at birth, for different regions (both sexes combined) [a, b]

Region	1950–1955	1980–1985	2020–2025
Northern America	69.0	74.6	79.7
Europe	65.3	73.2	79.1
Oceania	60.8	68.0	75.6
USSR	64.1	67.9	76.7
Latin America	51.2	64.5	72.8
Asia	41.1	59.3	72.8
Africa	38.0	49.9	65.2
Developed countries	65.7	72.3	78.7
Developing countries	41.0	57.6	70.4
World total	45.9	59.6	71.3

[a] In years, medium variant used for projection.
[b] Adapted from *World Population Prospects, 1988* (United Nations publication, Sales No. E.88.XIII.7), reference *12*, by kind permission of the publisher.

Table 7. Elderly population, aged 60 years or more, in millions by region (1950, 1985, and projections for 2025) [a]

Region	Total population 1985	Elderly population					
		1950		1985		2025 [b]	
		No.	%	No.	%	No.	%
Europe	492	51	12.9	88	17.8	138	27.0
Northern America	265	20	12.1	43	16.4	88	26.4
USSR	277	16	9.0	37	13.5	72	20.6
Oceania	25	1	11.3	3	12.3	7	18.5
Asia	2834	92	6.7	205	7.2	698	14.3
Latin America	404	9	5.3	27	6.8	97	12.7
Africa	557	12	5.4	27	4.9	101	6.4
Developed countries	1174	95	11.4	189	16.1	343	25.3
Developing countries	3680	106	6.3	243	6.6	858	12.1
World total	4854	201	8.0	432	8.9	1201	14.8

[a] Adapted from *World Population Prospects, 1988* (United Nations publication, Sales No. E.88.XIII.7), reference *12*, by kind permission of the publisher.
[b] Medium variant used for projection.

Table 8. Causes of death in 1980 in developed and developing countries, and world total [a]

Causes of death	Percentage of deaths		
	Developed countries	Developing countries	World total
Diseases of the circulatory system	54	19	26
Neoplasms	19	5	8
Infectious and parasitic diseases	8	40	33
Injury and poisoning	6	5	5
Perinatal mortality	2	8	6
All other causes	12	23	21

[a] Adapted from reference 13.

It is often assumed that chronic diseases develop as countries become more affluent. Although striking increases in deaths from these causes are evident between very poor countries and those with an average gross national product (GNP) of US$ 2000, the age-adjusted mortality of men and women aged 35–69 years of age, i.e., in an age span of potential economic activity, is dominated by cardiovascular disease and cancers in countries with a modest as well as a high GNP (Fig. 4). In countries with a GNP of US$ 3000–4000, the burden of cardiovascular disease and cancers is nearly as great as in the very affluent countries with an average income three times greater. Thus, modest increases in prosperity in populations with low GNP seem to be associated with the most marked increases in the proportion of these chronic diseases, which pose a major long-term burden on the health services of a country.

The link between increased economic development and the increased rates of cardiovascular diseases and cancers in the population is mediated by the acquisition of certain life-style characteristics. The changes in disease pattern are therefore not inevitable. Fig. 5 shows how the principal components of the diet tend to be related to a nation's relative affluence. As GNP increases, there is a progressive substitution of dietary fat from animal sources for complex carbohydrates. Free sugars, especially sucrose and glucose syrups, also form a much higher proportion of the total dietary carbohydrates in very affluent communities, e.g., 50% compared with the 5–10% observed in many communities with a low income. Thus, variation in the consumption of starchy foods and animal fats is the most striking feature of the different dietary patterns of societies with different degrees of affluence.

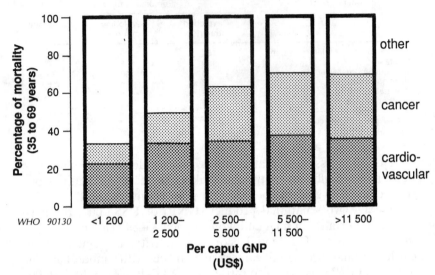

Fig. 4. Proportion of deaths from cardiovascular diseases, cancer, and other diseases, for both sexes aged 35–69, in relation to per caput gross national product[a]

[a] This diagram is based on an analysis of cause-specific mortality rates for the ages 35–69 years, from the WHO international mortality data base, adjusted to the world population, standard-age distribution. Fifty-two countries satisfied selection criteria for this analysis: information was available on national mortality by age group and on per capita gross national product (GNP), and the population numbered more than one million. Countries were divided into five groups according to GNP. Information on GNP was obtained from The World Bank (14).

Burkitt & Trowell (16), after reviewing the descriptive epidemiological data from many developing and developed countries, concluded that there is usually a sequence in the emergence of chronic disease as the diet of the developing country becomes more "westernized". Appendicitis and diabetes tend to occur early, followed after several decades by coronary heart disease and gallstones, then cancer of the large bowel, and finally various chronic disorders of the gastrointestinal tract.

Such changes have occurred more obviously in countries or population groups undergoing rapid transition between different cultural stages. For example, the Australian Aborigines traditionally derived most of their diet from roots and vegetables that contained much fibre. During the first half of the 20th century, white flour and sugar became their predominant sources of dietary carbohydrate, and this change, together with a sedentary life-style, was linked to

34

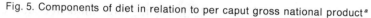

Fig. 5. Components of diet in relation to per caput gross national product[a]

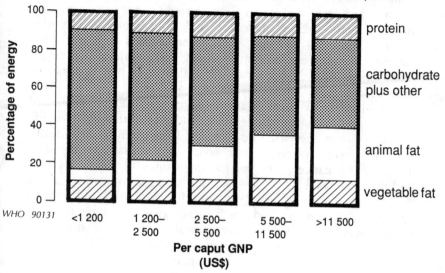

[a] This diagram is based on an analysis of diet components, GNP, and mortality rates. Fifty-two countries satisfied selection criteria for this analysis: information was available on per capita gross national product (GNP) and on energy and fat consumption, and the population numbered more than one million. Information on diet components was obtained from FAO (15), and on GNP from The World Bank (14).

the emergence of high rates of obesity and diabetes, followed by hypertension and coronary heart disease.

American Indians in the USA, who formerly consumed maize (corn) in large quantities, have experienced gross obesity and diabetes since changing their main sources of dietary carbohydrate to white flour and sugar. Now, more than 50% of Pima Indians over 35 years of age have diabetes. The dietary transition, and the associated obesity, appear to be important causes of the diabetes; however, other life-style changes, including reduced physical activity and increased stress, are possible contributors. Similarly, in the South Pacific Island of Nauru, 70% of people over the age of 50 years have diabetes. This change, which followed the rapid introduction of a cash income with a sedentary life-style, has produced a dramatic change in health.

The dietary staple in southern China has been rice for many centuries; in the north the main staple is corn or wheat. Traditionally, fat and sugar consumption has been low and animal protein consumption especially low. However, the diet is gradually changing in the cities to resemble that of the more affluent countries, and this has been associated with the appearance of significant coronary heart disease and diabetes. For example, in Shanghai County, China, during 1960–1962, cancer, cerebrovascular disease, and heart disease were the sixth, seventh, and eighth most common causes of mortality, whereas by 1978–1980 they had become the three leading causes of death (*17*).

The island of Mauritius, inhabited by one million people of various ethnic backgrounds, has experienced substantial gains in life expectancy over the past four decades. Concurrently, new health problems have emerged, and today cardiovascular diseases, diabetes, and cancers are the leading causes of morbidity and mortality. Deaths from cardiovascular diseases accounted for about 2% of all deaths in the early 1940s, and for about 45% of deaths in the 1980s. Age-standardized death rates, since 1960, have doubled for coronary heart disease, have remained high for stroke (in contrast to decreases in most other countries of the world), and have trebled for cancer of the breast in women.

Among the developing countries, Mauritius is frequently cited as an example of a country in which economic and social transition has occurred unusually rapidly. The emergence of chronic degenerative diseases associated with this transition has had serious implications for the direct costs to the health sector and, indirectly, to the national economy. The national government has, therefore, recently committed itself to a programme of developing "primordial",[1] primary, and secondary prevention strategies for the prevention and control of these recently acquired, diet-related diseases.

2.2.1 Urbanization, changing diet, and chronic diseases in developing countries

A striking change in developing countries has been the rapid increase in the proportion of people living in urban areas. This has had an immediate impact on the nature of the food supply, because no longer is a household relying on the ready availability of home-grown produce or on its storage within the household. The cash economy is of far greater significance for the urban household's food supply, and expanding urban communities place great demands on the transport and storage systems for food. Food preservation

---

[1] A primordial prevention strategy aims at preventing the emergence of predisposing conditions in communities in which they have not yet appeared.

therefore becomes of even greater significance than in the rural areas, and the availability of large numbers of people within a confined area provides a ready market for the development of small and medium-sized food industries. These developments are often encouraged by government subsidies, tax incentives, or administrative support as governments seek to solve the problem of both urban unemployment and food supply.

Not surprisingly, therefore, analyses of the dietary patterns of urban and rural dwellers in the same country show striking differences. There is an almost universal increase in fat and sugar consumption in urban areas compared with the related rural communities, which usually have to depend on their staple crops of cereals, tubers, vegetables, and fruits.

Thus, there are social and economic pressures for developing countries to change their diet towards that of affluent societies. As urban societies grow and generate money, they also perceive the new diet, similar to that of other affluent communities, as a symbol of their newly acquired status. They therefore tend to adopt diets containing more animal products, fats, and sugars. Within the urban setting, the food industry can also flourish and exert substantial influence by promoting the consumption of soft drinks, meat products, confectionery, snack foods, and other convenience foods rich in free sugars and fats. This commercial activity is rarely based on health considerations; the consequences for the health of consumers may often be detrimental.

As the urban elite (e.g., government civil servants and other professional groups) in the developing world experience higher rates of cardiovascular disease and cancers, there is an inevitable increase in the demand for medical therapy of the kind found in affluent societies. The provision of high-technology, hospital-based medical care within the cities of developing countries both distorts the pattern, and escalates the costs, of health care.

Hypertension and heart disease are already major health problems in many African cities and are of rapidly increasing concern in Asia. For example, the prevalence of high blood pressure in both men and women is at least four times as high in urban as in rural areas of Ghana (18). The transition from village to urban life-styles in Papua New Guinea, reviewed by Sinnett et al. (19), has been followed by increases in hospital admission rates for hypertension from 0.5 per 100 000 in 1961 to 7.5 per 100 000 in 1984. Hypertension was found especially in urbanized communities with long periods of European contact, together with obesity and maturity-onset diabetes. More recently, a significantly increased number of cases of coronary heart disease has been reported in Papua New Guinea.

Urban populations in Latin America have patterns of mortality, in persons surviving childhood, very similar to those of Europe and North America. A study of 12 cities (2 "western" and 10 Latin American) showed that in all the cities, whether "developed" or "developing", the leading causes of death after childhood were cardiovascular diseases and cancer.

Major differences are now emerging between the health patterns of urban and rural areas in the developing world. Statistics used for the disease patterns of the developing world markedly underestimate the current impact of cardiovascular disease and cancers in urban communities in Africa, Asia, the eastern Mediterranean region, and Latin America. Large increases in the urban population are expected, especially in developing countries (20), and, with these, a deterioration in many aspects of the nutritional quality of food is likely. This suggests that there is an urgent need to rethink national agricultural and food policies for urban as well as rural communities, before governments in developing countries are perhaps overwhelmed by the demands for diagnosis and management of diseases that can now be linked to current and projected dietary changes.

2.2.2 Trends in diet and chronic diseases in developed countries

In developed countries, diseases related to life-style (including diet, alcohol consumption, smoking, and the level of physical activity) account for most morbidity and mortality. Age-standardized mortality rates for cardiovascular disease and cancers vary considerably among, as well as within, countries, as do rates for non-insulin-dependent diabetes, liver cirrhosis, dental caries, and bone diseases. These differences can be related to differences in behaviour patterns and particularly to diet. In Belgium, for instance, regional differences in mortality from ischaemic heart disease and in liver cirrhosis show a clear correlation with regional differences in the fatty acid composition and the alcohol content of the diet, respectively.

Age-adjusted mortality rates from cardiovascular diseases and from certain cancers have changed significantly in developed countries but to very different degrees. For instance, changes in mortality from ischaemic heart disease in men aged 30–69 years between 1970 and 1985 ranged from −49% in the USA to +72% in Poland. Heterogeneous trends in mortality rates for cardiovascular disease in developed countries are largely unexplained in the absence of precise surveillance data on possible determinants. However, in some countries attempts have been made to explain the national changes. In the USA, the reduction in average blood cholesterol level was estimated to account for 30% of the decline in mortality rates for ischaemic heart disease (21). Taken as a whole, the evidence from comparisons among and within developed countries supports the view that a range of chronic diseases can be prevented to a substantial extent by life-style changes, among which diet plays a crucial role.

2.3 Changes in human dietary patterns: a longer-term view

2.3.1 An evolutionary and historical perspective

With changes in human culture and technology come changes in patterns of food production, processing, and storage. In addition, with increases in economic prosperity within populations (or segments of populations) come new consumer expectations and demands. Recent and continuing changes in diet in some developing countries resemble, to a variable extent, changes that have previously occurred in the diets of developed countries. A long-term historical view may help to set these changes in perspective.

2.3.2 Major historical changes leading to the "affluent" diet

The human diet has changed profoundly over what, in terms of the long and gradual process of human biological evolution, is a very short period of time. In most pre-agricultural societies, the supply of food was variable and uncertain, dependent on seasons, and often associated with periods of severe shortage or starvation. Deficiency diseases have been age-old companions of primitive and pre-industrialized societies. The human species is an unspecialized (omnivorous) eater, capable of surviving on a diet consisting mainly of meat, or one consisting almost entirely of vegetable matter (22). Anthropological studies of the diets of hunter-gatherer societies that have survived into the 20th century include that of the Bushmen of the Kalahari Desert in southern Africa, and provide a valuable evolutionary perspective on modern dietary practices in developed countries. The typical diet of most of today's surviving hunter-gatherers, living in relatively fertile areas of the world, consists mainly of a wide range of different foods of plant origin plus some meat, which makes up about one-quarter of the diet by weight. The anthropological studies indicate that the fat intake of prehistoric people living in temperate climates was about 20% of total calories (i.e., half the current intake in developed countries) with an appreciably higher ratio of unsaturated to saturated fatty acids. Fibre intake appears to have been about 45 grams per day, compared with 15 grams or less in present developed-country diets, and the intake of vitamin C was several times as high as that now observed in affluent societies. Assuming that the modern human species, *Homo sapiens*, evolved 30 000 to 50 000 years ago, then the species has subsisted for most of its history on low-fat, high-fibre diets, rich in vitamin C and many other micronutrients, to which it presumably adapted biologically to achieve optimum function. The profile of foods consumed by the hunter-gatherer persisted until the first agricultural revolution approximately 10 000 years ago.

2.3.3 *Agricultural revolutions*

A greatly improved food supply followed the cultivation of crops in the first agricultural revolution. Continuity of food supplies became more certain, although still subject to drought, pests and other natural hazards. This led to a better nutritional status, better resistance to infection, and lower mortality in infancy and childhood. As population numbers increased, so did the pressure on the food supply, and this sometimes led to undernutrition and a new rise in mortality from infection.

The second agricultural revolution, dating from the mid-18th century in Europe, led to an unprecedented abundance of food—assisted by the introduction of the energy-rich potato from America, of legumes, and, in southern Europe, of maize. Crop rotation, mixed farming, and finally mechanized farm implements were also very significant developments. These improvements were sufficient to feed populations that trebled in size between the end of the 17th century and the mid-19th century.

As with the first agricultural revolution, these developments were associated with population increases, reflecting particularly a fall in childhood mortality from infections, because of the improved nutritional status. The surplus population migrated to the cities and provided the work-force for the industrial revolution, but at the same time created a new pressure on food supplies. This provided a new impetus for technological developments in food processing, transport, and preservation.

Subsequently, in the second half of the 19th century, the "sanitary revolution" in Europe led to effective control of the waterborne diseases and some of the foodborne infectious diseases (e.g., typhoid fever). Nearly half of the fall in mortality from infectious diseases during those decades was attributable to reduced mortality from tuberculosis, due mainly to improvements in diet and housing; most of the rest was due to reduced mortality from typhus, other filth-related fevers, diarrhoea, dysentery, cholera, smallpox, and scarlet fever, in which an improved diet also played a significant role (23).

Concomitant with the increased production and the improved distribution of food were enormous technological changes in food processing. Also, edible plants and farm animals were improved by selective breeding. About 200 years ago, the Industrial Revolution also began to transform the life-styles of people in Western Europe and North America.

These agricultural and technological activities contributed to the development, in industrialized societies, of a modern diet that, in nutrient profile and energy content, is far removed from the diets of the hunter-gatherer and peasant-agriculture phases of human cultural evolution. In northern Europe and North America, these cumulative changes in diet have led to an increased supply of protein-rich foods, and also of saturated fatty acids, since animal storage fats are consumed in greater quantities, while the essential structural fatty acids found particularly in plants form a smaller part of the diet.

Fat intake rose steadily, fibre intake declined, and the consumption of free sugars rose as consumption of complex carbohydrates fell. The energy density of food has therefore increased in recent centuries, at a time when human energy expenditure (physical activity) has declined. Comparison between the diet of the late-Paleolithic time (Stone Age) and the current American diet shows large changes in protein, fat, sodium, potassium, and calcium intake (24).

Today, therefore, the human diet of developed countries is very different from that of about 150 generations ago, when the human species lived on wild plants and animals. Even 10 generations ago, before the Industrial Revolution, diets were different. The most significant changes in the human diet have, in fact, taken place only during the last few centuries, and the human species has had virtually no time to adapt biologically to the rapid changes in the types and amounts of food available.

Table 9 gives figures for the United Kingdom that highlight some of the major dietary changes that have occurred over the last 200 years. The striking change is the substantial decline in the intake of complex carbohydrates accompanied by the progressive rise in fat and sugar consumption. These changes over a 200-year period are mimicked in many ways by the differences found today between the dietary patterns of hunter-gatherers and peasant agriculturalists in developing countries and of people in developed countries, which are illustrated in Fig. 6.

Recent approaches to nutrition in Europe and North America

In the 1930s, the primary concern in Europe and North America was the elimination of deficiency diseases, and the widely promoted concept of a "balanced diet" arose from efforts to prevent these. This concept was based on the recognition that an appropriate mixture of food items would provide the minimum requirement of protein, vitamins, and minerals needed by the body. By the late 1950s, epidemiological research had begun to indicate that some chronic diseases that were not normally associated with undernutrition might nevertheless also be nutrition-related. Nutritional excess (or "overnutrition"), in parallel with nutritional deficiencies (e.g., of iodine and iron), thus became a focus of research. Since then, cumulative scientific evidence has confirmed and elaborated the role of diet in the development of many of these chronic diseases.

Table 9. Estimated per caput consumption in the United Kingdom of various foodstuffs, 1770, 1870, 1970[a]

Foodstuff	Grams per person per day		
	1770	1870	1970
Fat	25	75	145
Sugar	10	80	150
Potatoes	120	400	240
Wheat flour	500	375	200
Cereal crude fibre	5	1	0.2

[a] Reproduced from reference *16*, by kind permission of the publisher.

Fig. 6. Percentage of energy obtained from different food components and salt and fibre intakes of different human groups [a]

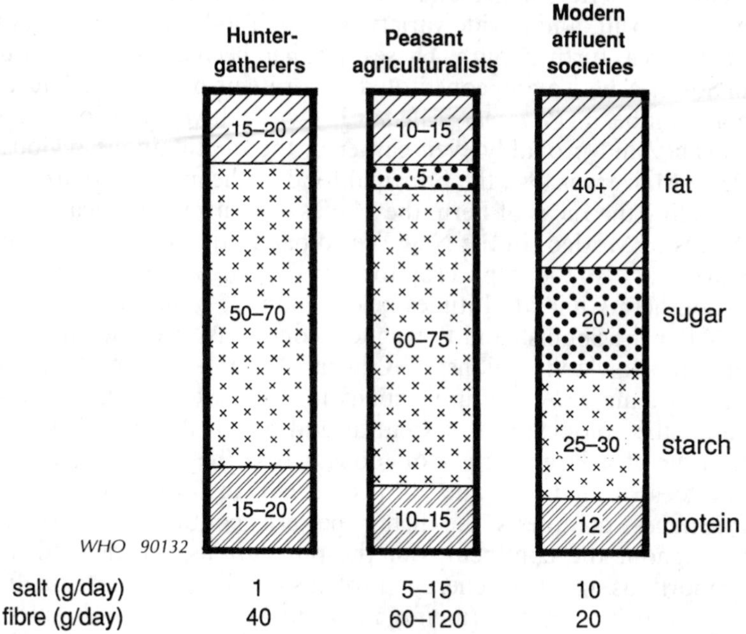

	Hunter-gatherers	Peasant agriculturalists	Modern affluent societies	
fat	15–20	10–15	40+	
	x 50–70 x	5	20	sugar
		60–75	25–30	starch
protein	15–20	10–15	12	

WHO 90132

	Hunter-gatherers	Peasant agriculturalists	Modern affluent societies
salt (g/day)	1	5–15	10
fibre (g/day)	40	60–120	20

[a] Reproduced from reference 25, by kind permission of the publisher, with slight modifications.

Thus, the concepts of the requirements for a balanced diet in developed countries have, in recent decades, changed radically from the needs recognized earlier this century, and are very different from those in preceding centuries. These new concepts are now becoming as relevant to developing countries as to developed countries.

2.3.4 Dietary change in Latin America

The native populations of Latin America have traditionally been agriculturalists with a wide variety of diets. Thus, before countries were governed by the Spanish and Portuguese there were diverse indigenous patterns of agriculture with, for example, potatoes, beans, and guinea-pigs forming the main dietary items in the highland regions of South America. Camelids, for example the llama and alpaca, were also a substantial source of meat and milk in

Bolivia, Chile, and Peru, as well as serving as beasts of burden and providing wool for clothing. In Mexico and in the northern parts of Central America, maize and red beans were the staple crops, with cassava, fruit, and a wide variety of other foods being grown in the jungle areas further south. These crops had been grown for centuries in South America and constituted major items of the diet. Thus, the common bean (*Phaseolus vulgaris* L.) was cultivated as long ago as 5000 BC, and probably even earlier in the mountainous regions of Peru. Maize was also the principal food of the ancient civilizations, including the Incas of Peru, the Mayas of Central America, and the Aztecs of Mexico. In the New World before the time of Columbus, maize was also the staple crop for a whole range of people who lived in southern Chile at altitudes below about 3300 metres.

After the Spanish and Portuguese conquests, rice was introduced into the lowland regions of Central America and cattle-rearing became a major agricultural activity in South America. On the other hand, the colonization of Central and South America led to the transfer of a large variety of foods across the world, e.g., maize, potatoes, tomatoes, and beans. Following the Spanish and Portuguese conquests, the dietary patterns continued to be diverse throughout the continent, but the populations still derived large proportions of their energy, proteins, and micronutrients from staples such as cereals (mainly maize in Mexico, Central America, and the tropical and subtropical regions of South America, rice in some parts of Central and South America, and wheat in northern Mexico and the southern segment of South America), legumes (black, red, or white beans in most of the continent) and tubers (potatoes in Andean regions and yams in northeastern Brazil). Other vegetables and a wide variety of fruits were available, but they were not eaten regularly in large amounts by most populations. Cane sugar was introduced as a cash crop and sugar has become a major source of dietary energy in several Latin American countries. Poultry, eggs and, to a smaller extent, pork, are now the most common foods of animal origin, although intake is relatively low. Cattle, although raised for export of meat in many countries, provide meat as a major food only in Argentina, southern Brazil, Uruguay, and the more affluent groups in other countries. Fish is not a common food, even in coastal areas and around the rivers and lakes.

Many diets are based on the habitual consumption of a few foods that supply most of the nutrients and dietary energy (for example, the maize-and-beans food system of southern Mexico and Guatemala, or the yam-and-beans system of northeastern Brazil). These monotonous diets favour the development of specific nutrient deficiencies, e.g., of iron and vitamin A, and make it difficult, though not impossible, to satisfy the populations' energy and protein needs, especially in the case of young children.

South America is now seeing very substantial changes in diet, as urban communities grow and the patterns of demand influence the transport and sale of food; in most countries, 50–70% of the population still live in rural areas, and consume mainly cereals, legumes (beans) and other vegetables, with few animal foods. In Argentina, southern Brazil, and Uruguay, a special situation exists, the diet of large segments of the population being based on beef. Whereas subsistence farmers in the country continue to grow much of what they eat, city-dwellers rely on diets based on cereals or fibres and legumes, but these diets are rapidly changing to resemble more closely the North American and Western European diets. Processed and semi-processed foods have supplanted many staples, especially in urban and suburban areas. Aggressive commercial publicity and the impact of films, television, and magazines, which depict certain foods and beverages as being linked to higher social status, have increased the use of products with little or no nutritional value. These foods, rich in fat and sugar, have become important socially if not as yet in nutritional terms, and are now beginning to be substituted for the better traditional foods.

In the wake of urbanization, urban slums have emerged, resulting in drastic changes in food habits. The diet of slum-dwellers is of poor quality: legume consumption has decreased and malnutrition increased; some processed foods have been incorporated. The urban middle-income groups depend on local and processed foods containing more fats and free sugars, as well as more animal foods than rural diets. The higher-income groups have dietary patterns similar to North American or Western European diets, with relatively high consumption of animal foods, vegetable fats, and sugars. Smoking and the consumption of carbonated sugar-containing beverages and of alcohol are common in most countries. In general, physical activity has decreased as a result of urbanization among men, women, children of school age, and adolescents.

The food industry has also developed, and now has better means of communication and systems for the commercial distribution of foods. Better sources of proteins and micronutrients, as well as more hygienic foods, have been introduced as a result, but an undesirable increase in the intake of fats, refined carbohydrates, and salt is also occurring.

With these rapid changes in the urban diet have come further problems of malnutrition in the last decade as a result of the economic crises that have affected most Latin American countries. These have forced the lower-income groups to replace some of the more expensive staples (e.g., animal foods and legumes) by cheaper, and often less nutritious, products.

The introduction of the African palm to South America as a source of oil has proved to be economically attractive. Production of the palm oil is increasing in many Latin American countries, and in some, such as Costa Rica and Venezuela, it is already a major source of dietary fat for the population.

2.3.5 *Dietary change in Africa*

The dietary patterns found in Africa have, for centuries, differed from country to country and region to region, with large differences in agricultural practices in the north, south, east, and west. The main dietary changes in Africa followed the slave trade and colonization —at the end of the 19th and the beginning of the 20th century. The development of an export trade in cash crops, such as cocoa, rubber, cotton, coffee, and sisal, meant that most of the good land was given over to cash crops. Food crops were grown only on the marginal and poor soils. High prices for cash crops and minerals—including petroleum—made it easier to import wheat, rice, and even beef from outside the continent. Analyses of the effects of cash-cropping on the dietary patterns and nutritional state of the people provide a very mixed picture. In some cases, cash-cropping has been disastrous, with a marked increase in the area of arid land (for example, in the sub-Saharan belt); but elsewhere, cash-cropping has been an effective way of increasing the food security of a region.

One of the major features of the social development of Africa is the very rapid increase in the population. High birth rates have meant that the population structure is dominated by a very high proportion of children. The increase in mouths to feed is now putting a great strain on food resources.

The production of local cereals and plant products like sorghum, millet, maize, yam, and plantain cannot keep up with the rising population, and cassava (which will grow on poor soil) has become more and more important. In the rural areas, local food production on the marginal land cannot support the population explosion. Energy and protein insufficiency are common, while nutrient deficiencies are still seen. Since 1970, drought and other natural catastrophes have resulted in undernutrition or famine in more than 20 countries. This situation highlights the precarious food-supply situation in Africa.

The development programmes of most African countries include the promotion of greater reliance on locally produced foods and on greatly reduced importation of exotic, highly refined foods. Economic stresses, particularly in the present decade, have brought widespread dietary hardship and restrictions, especially among the lower-income populations in and around urban areas.

The process of urbanization in Africa can be exemplified by what has happened in the United Republic of Tanzania and Zimbabwe over the last 20 years. Traditionally, the population is agriculture-based, living in rural areas and consuming a home-produced cereal-based diet. Even today, 80% of the population live in the rural areas. Maize, rice, millet, and wheat, along with local meat, bananas, beans, green vegetables, and yams, could provide an adequately mixed traditional diet. Economic development over the past two decades has resulted in an overall increase in purchasing power and has brought about dietary behavioural changes in all segments of the population. This has resulted in three distinct population subgroups: rural, urban, and urban slum-dwellers.

The rural population has maintained the traditional diet, but total food intake, including fat, has increased. With increases in commerce, mining, and other industries, the population migration from rural to urban areas has generated the urban slums, whose residents are facing very serious dietary and nutritional inadequacy. Lack of physical exercise is resulting in obesity among non-working females of this subgroup. The urban elite, in contrast, though a small fraction, have drastically altered their food habits, influenced both by local and international food industries, and now tend to consume high-fat, energy-rich, high-salt, and processed sugar-based items. Soft drinks, alcohol, and ready-to-eat food items are popular, thus disturbing the traditional home-based diets. No special nutritional programmes are in operation in urban areas. Stroke, coronary heart disease, diabetes, and other diseases of affluence are increasing in this group. Thus the dual problems of undernutrition and overnutrition have emerged in the urban context, the latter tending to increase the occurrence of chronic diseases among the urban elite population.

Some of the countries in the African region have now developed their own food and nutrition policies. Most of these aim to eradicate malnutrition, but it is important to maintain awareness of the emergence of overnutrition and its resultant effect on chronic diseases. This awareness should not be limited to the urban elite, but should encompass the emerging affluent commercial/business sector in rural areas and small towns.

2.3.6 Dietary change in China

In all countries, dietary patterns change with socioeconomic development. In ancient China, as a result of the great disparity in socioeconomic situation between the feudal nobles and the common people, a basic dietary pattern of high-cereal, high-vegetable intake had developed for the common people, while, at the same time, a different cereal-based dietary pattern, high in meat and fish, existed for the rich. About 2000 years ago, Confucius taught his students: "The higher the quality of foods the better, and never rely upon the delicacy of cooking". Consequently, the concept of enjoying a diet high in animal food, and a preference for meat and greasy foods, have been shaped over hundreds of years. So, in the earliest medical classics, a dietary guideline based on experience was given as: "Cereals—the basic, fruits—the subsidiary, meat—the beneficial, vegetables—the supplementary", which gives a hint of the prevalent dietary problems from the medical point of view.

Since the founding of the People's Republic of China, social change and intensive preventive activities have made tremendous progress in controlling infectious and parasitic diseases. Consequently, annual population mortality rates have decreased to 6–7 per thousand and life expectancy has increased to 68 years. Food security policies have been established that assure the basic needs in staple foods and edible oil for the whole urban and rural population.

Economic reform and the new policy for agriculture over the past 10 years have accelerated agricultural and industrial development, resulting in widespread food adequacy and increased per caput income. There has been a rapid increase in the consumption of foods of animal origin from 26.5 kg/year per caput in 1957 to 47.7 kg/year in 1984. Oil intake has also increased as a result of excellent harvests of oil-seed crops. Thus, the national dietary pattern is moving towards larger quantities of animal food, higher fat intake, and smaller quantities of cereals.

The process of urbanization in China has been slower than in other developing countries because of official policy; 75% of the population are now in rural areas. Owing to the increase in agricultural production and the doubled or tripled average income, the diet in rural areas has been changing towards higher meat and fat intakes—but it is still basically a cereal-based diet. In large cities such as Beijing and Tianjin, the trend to high consumption of meat and fat has been marked, with 30% of energy being derived from fat.

2.3.7 *Dietary change in India*

Over time, traditional regional diets have emerged in India, and these have been based primarily on local agricultural practices, climate, and religious beliefs. Despite many centuries of cultural invasions, traditional diets remained unchanged, although some newer dietary habits were added. Diets were usually carefully prescribed in many parts of India to suit occupation, health and physiological status, and the amount of physical activity. Times for eating were prescribed, overeating was prohibited, and vegetarian diets were recommended. Until recently, locally grown agricultural products have dominated diets in India, thus creating distinct rice-based, wheat-based, and millet-based diets.

Because of religious traditions and taboos, the inclusion of meat, especially pork, in the diet remains very limited. In recent decades, developments in food storage and distribution systems have resulted in the ability to move food grain to different parts of the country, and cultural interactions have further modified the typical regional diets. Nevertheless, the majority of the population continue to eat a cereal-based diet.

Gopalan (*26*) stated that the important dietary changes that take place as Indian populations move up the socioeconomic scale appear to be:

1. An increased intake of legumes, vegetables, milk and, in case of non-vegetarians, foods of animal origin—changes that may be considered beneficial from the nutritional point of view.
2. Substitution of millet (coarse grain) by the more prestigious cereals, wheat and rice, with a progressively increasing preference for the highly polished varieties of rice with increasing socioeconomic advancement. This change is usually accompanied

by a reduction in the overall cereal intake (though cereal intake continues to be relatively high by European and North American standards, even in the most affluent Indian groups).These changes have resulted in a decrease in the overall fibre content of the diet. The total substitution of millet by polished rice or refined wheat results in a reduction in the fibre content of the diet of more than 50%.

3. Progressive increases in the intake of edible fat, with increasing preference for hydrogenated fats in the place of vegetable oils (in the case of the middle classes) and, in the most prosperous segments, a relatively high intake of ghee (clarified butter). The diet of nearly 17% of the rural poor does not include any edible oil, whereas fat intake in the diet of the top-income bracket in the country could provide over 30% of the energy in the diet. The distribution of fat intakes in Indian populations is highly skewed, with about 5% of the population consuming nearly 40% of the available fat.

4. Increased intake of sugar and sweets (which the poor can hardly afford).

5. Increase in the overall energy intake in relation to energy expenditure—leading to obesity.

The "invisible" fat intake in the diets of even poor Indians ranges from 20 to 50 g daily. The linoleic acid derived from "invisible" fat contributes an average of 4.8–7.0% of the dietary energy. Even poor Indian diets are reasonably adequate in fat.

During the last three decades, increases in urbanization, and the availability of cafeteria or hotel-based meals in the cities and towns explain these dramatic changes in the long-standing cultural dietary habits. Tea, coffee, soft drinks, and snacks are now also consumed widely among both the middle-income and the poorer segments of the population. Smoking and alcohol consumption have increased in many population groups. Physical exercise has decreased among the urban populations, contributing to obesity.

2.3.8 *Dietary change in Japan*

Japan was relatively isolated from Western influences until the latter half of the 19th century. It was a feudal society in which the average person's diet was low in food and nutrients (Table 10). Changes in the diet were relatively small until after the Second World War.

Table 10. Changes in daily per caput intakes of nutrients and major groups of foods in Japan, 1850–1987

Nutrient/Food	1850[a]	1952[b]	1980[b]	1987[b]
Energy (kcal$_{th}$)	< 1800	2109	2119	2075
Protein (g)	< 50	70.0	78.7	78.9
Animal protein (g)	< 20	22.6	39.2	40.1
Total fat (g)	< 10	20.1	55.6	56.6
Animal fat (g)	< 5	7.0	26.9	27.9
Carbohydrate (g)	< 380	412	309	295
Rice (g)	< 350	352	225	212
Meat (g)	< 5	10.6	17.9	70.8
Milk (g)	0	10.6	115.2	117.9
Fish (g)	< 60	82.3	92.5	90.5

[a] From an old book referring to the Edo area.
[b] Ministry of Health and Welfare of Japan, National Nutrition Survey.

The Japanese Ministry of Health and Welfare has conducted National Nutrition Surveys every year since 1946. There have been large increases in meat and fat consumption. The average energy intake derived from fat has increased each year and reached 24% in 1980. Intakes of rice fell substantially during the 1960s and 1970s with a marked increase in fruit consumption as well as in milk intake. In 1988, 15.3% of energy consumed came from protein and 59.9% from carbohydrate. Intakes of dietary fat, saturated fat, cholesterol, sugar, dietary fibre, and protein are all at present estimated to be within acceptable limits. Salt intake is an exception, but has been falling progressively and had reached a value of 12.3 g per person per day in 1982. Although in recent years the average intake of calcium has been slightly less than recommended, intakes of the other nutrients have been estimated to exceed the recommended daily allowance.

The well recognized secular increase in the growth rates of Japanese children seems to be closely linked to the intake of dietary protein, particularly from animal sources. The population over 65 years of age is now rapidly increasing and it is predicted that more than one in five persons will be over 65 years of age by 2020. These changes in life expectancy reflect improvements in diet and a reduction in premature mortality from pneumonia, bronchitis, and tuberculosis since the end of the Second World War, with a later decline in mortality from cerebrovascular disease. There has been a progressive increase in mortality from cancer, diabetes, and heart disease. These adverse developments led the Japanese Dietetic Association in 1984 to call for the development of dietary guidelines and nutrition policies in Japan (27). They noted the adverse trends in fat consumption and the very large variations in the eating habits of different families. They proposed the avoidance of excess intakes of salt, fat, and energy and promoted an increase in the consumption of unrefined cereals, vegetables, legumes, mushrooms, and seaweeds. They proposed a fat intake, for individuals, of 20–25% of energy with a very low content of saturated fatty acids; the polyunsaturated fatty acids, derived particularly from fish, should be half of the total fat intake.

Thus, the Association recognized the need to reverse some of the current trends in the food habits of the Japanese. Priority policies supporting activities for the improvement of nutritional status in Japan are as follows:

1. Nutrition survey system—conducted annually by the Ministry of Health and Welfare.
2. Nutrition education system, including school lunches.
3. Health care system—there are more than 10 000 hospitals (more than 20 beds) and 850 health centres in Japan.
4. Cooperation of the food industries. For example, tasty low-fat "hamburgers" are made from soya-bean protein and distributed for school lunches.

3. A SUMMARY OF THE RELATIONSHIPS BETWEEN DIET AND CHRONIC DISEASES

Given the extensive medical research over the last four decades into the link between diet and chronic disease, only a brief overview of the evidence is possible and readers are advised to consult the references cited, and previous WHO reports dealing with individual diseases, for a more detailed exposition.

3.1 Nature of research and evidence used

The evidence relating diet to chronic diseases comes from epidemiological investigations and from controlled trials in human beings. Laboratory experiments on animals and *in vitro* tests on tissues have also contributed to an understanding of the relationships between diet and the various chronic diseases described in this section. The links have been established on the basis of data from all these sources, and the analysis takes into account the strengths and weaknesses of the different types of study.

Descriptive epidemiological investigations of the relation between dietary factors and chronic diseases have yielded important hypotheses and valuable data, but they cannot be used alone to establish causality or to estimate the strength of the association between diet and diseases. Analytical epidemiological studies, such as cohort studies and case-control studies that compare information from sets of individuals within a population, usually provide more accurate estimates of such associations. The most consistent correlations between diet and chronic diseases have been obtained from comparisons of populations or population subgroups with substantially different dietary habits. In contrast, it is often more difficult to identify a diet–disease association within a population where the diets of the individual members are fairly homogeneous.

While the epidemiological evidence depends on observations made in whole populations or population subgroups, every population consists of individuals who may vary in their susceptibility to each disease. Part of this difference in susceptibility occurs for genetic reasons. As the dietary or social conditions within a population change in the direction that increases the risk of a specific disease, so an increasing proportion of individuals, particularly those who are most susceptible, develop the disease. For researchers, an important consequence of this inter-individual variability in susceptibility to disease is that some diet–disease relationships are difficult to identify within a single population, even though diet may strongly influence the average risk of disease occurrence within that population as a whole. In that case, the diet–disease relationship may be most evident in comparisons between populations that have different average (per caput) dietary intakes.

In controlled trials and experimental clinical studies, long exposure is usually required for the effect of a diet on the risk of chronic disease to become evident. Furthermore, it may be necessary to have strict selection criteria for participants in such studies in order to show an effect with small numbers in a reasonable time. This selection process may result in restricted and homogeneous study samples, which then may limit the applicability of results to the general population. Despite the limitations of the various types of study in human beings, repeated and consistent findings of an association between specific dietary factors and a disease suggest that such associations are real and indicative of a cause-and-effect relationship.

Experimental studies on animals make it possible to investigate more closely the links between diet and disease. However, extrapolation of data from animal studies to human beings is restricted by the limitations of animal models in simulating human diseases and human diets, and by differences in absorption and in metabolic processes among species. Thus, more confidence might be placed in data derived from studies on more than one animal species or test system, on results that have been reproduced in different laboratories, and on data that indicate a dose–response relationship.

Therefore, in addition to considering the strengths and weaknesses of each kind of study discussed above, and placing most confidence in data from studies on human beings, the significance and consistency of the data and the agreement between epidemiological, clinical, and laboratory evidence need to be taken into account in reaching conclusions about the influence of diet on the occurrence of chronic diseases.

3.2 Cardiovascular diseases

The most frequent cardiovascular diseases are obliterative atherosclerosis, arterial thrombosis, and hypertension. Each may be influenced by diet. Most evidence from studies in human beings relates to the effect of dietary variables on lipid and lipoprotein fractions, especially total and low-density lipoprotein cholesterol. The following section deals mainly with the relations between different dietary variables and serum total cholesterol, and with the relation between serum total cholesterol and the risk of coronary heart disease. The relation between high blood pressure and cerebrovascular disease will also be discussed.

3.2.1 *Coronary heart disease*

Coronary heart disease (CHD) as a public health problem became evident in Europe and North America early in this century. By the 1950s it had become the single major cause of adult death, and suspicions then began to emerge as to its likely causes. The approximately fivefold difference in rates among various developed countries (e.g., Finland compared with Japan) and the intrapopulation variation in rates, by socioeconomic class, ethnicity, and geographical location, emphasized the environmental basis of the condition. Further evidence for environmental determinants comes from the marked shifts in CHD rates seen in migrant populations that move across a geographical gradient in CHD risk and change their life-style.

On the cross-cultural level, the relation between diet and CHD was supported by the results of the Seven Countries Study (28, 29). In the seven countries, saturated fat intake varied between 3% of total energy in Japan and 22% in eastern Finland. Average serum total cholesterol values in these populations amounted to 4.3 mmol/l (165 mg/dl) in Japan and 7.0 mmol/l (270 mg/dl) in eastern Finland. The 15-year CHD incidence rates varied between 144 per 10 000 in Japan and 1202 per 10 000 in eastern Finland. The results suggested that, on a population level, serum total cholesterol was strongly related to the incidence of CHD. A strong correlation was also observed between the intake of saturated fat and serum total cholesterol, suggesting that the variation in serum total cholesterol level between populations could be largely explained by differences in saturated fat intake.

On a population basis, the risk of CHD rises progressively with increases in serum total cholesterol from 3.89 mmol/l (150 mg/dl). For many countries the whole population may be described as being at high risk. Studies in rural parts of China indicate an average total cholesterol level of 3.24 mmol/l (125 mg/dl) and this population has an incidence of CHD of only 4% of that observed in Great Britain. The concept of a "normal" total cholesterol, therefore, has little meaning; observational studies suggest that one population with an average total cholesterol level 10% lower than that of another will have one-third less CHD, and a 30% difference in total cholesterol predicts a fourfold difference in CHD.

The Seven Countries Study showed a strong positive relation between saturated fat intake and the 10-year incidence of CHD (30). There was some suggestion of a curvilinear relationship in these data, which became clearer when the follow-up period was extended to 20 years. Populations with an average saturated fat intake between 3% and 10% of energy intake were characterized by a serum total cholesterol level below 5.17 mmol/l (200 mg/dl) and by low mortality rates from CHD. When saturated fat intake was greater than 10% of energy intake a marked and progressive increase in CHD mortality was observed.

The role of different unsaturated fatty acids, e.g., mono-unsaturated and n–3 and n–6 polyunsaturated fatty acids, in the prevention of CHD remains unclear. Populations in some Mediterranean countries with a high intake of total fat (more than 40% of energy) derived predominantly from mono-unsaturated fatty acids (olive oil) have low rates of CHD. Eskimos, who also have a diet high in total fat and in n–3 polyunsaturated fatty acids, mainly derived from marine foods, also have low CHD rates. The diets of these populations are also, however, characterized by a low intake of saturated fatty acids. This may explain their low CHD rates. Populations with a long-standing intake of n–6 polyunsaturated fatty acids above 7% of energy do not exist. Therefore, information on the public health consequences of diets with amounts of n–6 polyunsaturated fatty acids above this level is not available.

Epidemiological studies carried out on middle-aged men provide clear evidence that the risk of CHD in individuals is increased by three major factors: high serum total cholesterol, high blood pressure, and cigarette smoking (31). There is also synergism between the risk factors, i.e., the presence of several risk factors, simultaneously, increases the risk of the disease more than would be expected from the sum of the individual risk factors. The fundamental importance of diet in the development of coronary heart disease is mediated through its effects on the development of hypercholesterolaemia and hypertension. Body-weight changes induced by changes in diet and physical activity are strongly related to changes in serum total cholesterol and blood pressure, and obesity is strongly related to diabetes, which is a further risk factor for CHD.

Several prospective studies have shown an inverse relation between high-density lipoprotein cholesterol and CHD incidence. Several negative correlates of high-density lipoprotein cholesterol have also been identified, e.g., overweight, alcohol abstention, smoking, and physical inactivity. This form of cholesterol seems, however, not to play an important role in explaining differences in CHD mortality between populations, and its dietary determinants will therefore not be discussed.

There has been substantial experimental work relating change in dietary lipid components to serum total cholesterol response. Although the earlier studies related dietary change to serum total cholesterol, it is now accepted that total cholesterol is an indicator of the atherogenic low-density lipoprotein fraction. Early work suggested that saturated fatty acids elevate serum cholesterol while polyunsaturated fatty acids reduce the level; mono-unsaturated fatty acids tended to have little direct effect but the relationship does not hold for all individual fatty acids, or necessarily for all isomers of the fatty acids (e.g., the *trans* fatty acids). However, saturated fatty acids with 12–16 carbon atoms have been found consistently to elevate serum levels of low-density lipoprotein cholesterol, and dietary cholesterol itself has predictable effects on serum cholesterol at very low intakes. Major individual variations in responsiveness were also evident.

Other dietary components, such as dietary fibre, have an effect on serum cholesterol in experimental studies and are correlated in intercountry comparisons. As with the fatty acids, the different forms of dietary fibre may have different effects on serum cholesterol. The dietary factors that affect serum cholesterol in a similar way tend to cluster together in many diets. Thus, as one compares national diets rich in foods of animal origin and refined cereals with a more "vegetarian" diet typical of many developing countries, the total fat, saturated fat, and cholesterol contents are greater, the content of polyunsaturated fatty acids, as a proportion of total fat, tends to be less, and the dietary fibre content also tends to be less. Since all these factors can affect serum cholesterol, their combined effects may be important in modifying the rate of progression of atherosclerosis. These concordant trends in diet also make it difficult to assess quantitatively the effects of the individual factors on the atherosclerosis process.

Population subgroups consuming diets rich in plant foods have lower CHD rates than the general population. For example, Seventh-Day Adventists in the Netherlands and Norway have CHD rates that are one-third to one-half of those in the general population. Californian Seventh-Day Adventists who eat meat have higher rates than do those who are vegetarians, and British vegetarians have a 30% lower rate of CHD mortality than non-vegetarians once an allowance is made for their lower rates of cigarette smoking. Serum cholesterol levels among vegetarians are significantly lower than among lacto-ovo-vegetarians and non-vegetarians.

Alcohol consumption also influences the occurrence of CHD. A slightly lower risk of CHD in light-to-moderate drinkers than in abstainers was shown in a number of observational studies in Israel, Scotland, the USA, and Yugoslavia. However, a recent study from the United Kingdom suggests that this association can be partly or wholly explained by the inclusion in the group of abstainers of ex-drinkers who had stopped drinking for health reasons (*32*). Alcohol ingestion does cause a favourable rise in the anti-atherogenic high-density lipoprotein fraction, but many epidemiological studies show that moderate and heavy drinkers have higher blood pressures than non-drinkers, and that abstinence from alcohol is followed by a fall in blood pressure.

Controlled trials in human beings using diet or drugs to reduce serum cholesterol show a reduction in the incidence and progression of CHD. Two carefully organized trials for the primary prevention of CHD, based only on dietary changes, showed that changing from a high to a low intake of saturated fats and replacing the fat with *n*–6 polyunsaturated fatty acids (such as linoleic acid) reduced serum cholesterol by 15% and led to a reduction of CHD incidence (*33, 34*).

Experimental studies showed an independent effect of dietary cholesterol on serum total cholesterol. This effect is smaller than that of saturated fatty acids. In several prospective cohort studies, an independent effect of dietary cholesterol on CHD incidence can be observed, a change of 200 mg of dietary cholesterol per 1000 kcal$_{th}$ (or 4.184 MJ) being associated with a 30% change in CHD incidence (*35*). Dietary cholesterol therefore contributes to CHD risk, and a population average intake of less than 300 mg/day has been recommended by most international committees.

A low intake of saturated fatty acids is the preferred option for preventing coronary heart disease and is the strategy that is still accepted by numerous international committees. In most developed countries, a high total fat intake coincides with a high saturated fat intake—diets with 40% of energy from total fat often provide 15–20% of the energy from saturated fat. Reducing total fat intake to 30% of energy will therefore have a substantial effect on saturated fatty acid intake in those populations, but should still allow the different unsaturated fatty acids to contribute up to 20% of energy. An FAO/WHO expert group concerned with dietary fats and oils in human nutrition recommended that 3% of energy should be taken as the lower limit for the essential fatty acid content of the diet (*36*).

3.2.2 *High blood pressure and cerebrovascular disease*

The topic of high blood pressure and cerebrovascular disease has been dealt with more extensively in previous WHO publications (*30,*

37–40), but recent analyses reinforce the need for preventive measures to limit the development of hypertension. The risk of both CHD and stroke increases progressively throughout the observed range of blood pressure (see Fig. 7) with an impressive consistency of data in each of nine major studies conducted in a number of different countries. When all the data are combined in a statistically appropriate manner, it is clear that there is a fivefold difference in CHD and a tenfold difference in risk of stroke over a range of diastolic blood pressure of 40 mmHg (5.33 kPa). Observational studies, when combined, show that a sustained difference of only 7.5 mmHg (1.0 kPa) in the diastolic blood pressure confers up to a 28% difference in risk of CHD and a 44% difference in the risk of stroke. Since in many developed countries, the risk of CHD may be three to six times that of stroke, the population benefit of a lower blood pressure will have its greatest impact by reducing the number of cases of CHD.

The combined results of therapeutic trials of drug therapy used to lower blood pressure provide data on 37 000 patients and show (Fig. 8) a marked reduction in the incidence of stroke, but a lower-

Fig. 7. Association between usual diastolic blood pressure (DBP) and risk of stroke and coronary heart disease [a, b]

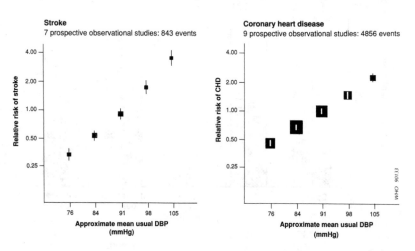

[a] The size of the boxes is proportional to the amount of information in each DBP category. The vertical lines denote 95% confidence limits. Values for mean usual DBP were estimated from later remeasurements in the Framingham study.
[b] Reproduced from reference *41*, by kind permission of the publisher.

than-expected effect in lowering the incidence of CHD. Diuretics were used in several of the trials and these drugs increase plasma cholesterol by 3–5%, which in turn would be expected to increase CHD rates by 5–10%. The benefits of lowering blood pressure are clear in both primary and secondary preventive trials, and there is no threshold below which a further lowering of blood pressure is without effect. One would therefore expect a primary preventive approach to be of major benefit since dietary manipulations, e.g., to reduce weight and restrict alcohol intake, have well recognized effects in lowering blood pressure. Some individuals also seem to benefit from a lower salt intake.

A recent large-scale multinational study (the Intersalt Study), involving 52 centres in 32 countries around the world, assessed the role of obesity, alcohol, and mineral intake in determining the progressive rise in blood pressure seen with age in most countries. A

Fig. 8. The overall effect of drug therapy in lowering high blood pressure in randomized trials on 37 000 subjects[a]

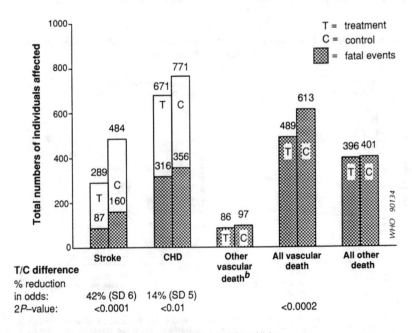

[a] Reproduced from reference 42, by kind permission of the publisher.
[b] Excludes death from stroke or CHD but includes death from unknown causes.

60

high body-mass index[1] and high alcohol intake had strong, independent effects on blood pressure. Salt (sodium chloride) intake (assessed from a single 24-h urine collection) had a weaker but significant effect on the rise in blood pressure with age. In the four populations with a particularly low salt intake of below 3 g/day, no increase of blood pressure with age was observed, but a salt intake of 6 g/day may be a more reasonable estimate of a safe upper limit. Other minerals measured, e.g., potassium and magnesium, seemed to play a role in limiting the rise of blood pressure and are readily found in diets rich in complex carbohydrates, which also contain a variety of other minerals that were not studied (*11*). Some, but not all, cross-sectional and intervention studies suggest a beneficial effect of calcium intake on blood pressure, but at the moment there is not enough evidence to justify a recommendation for an increased calcium intake. Epidemiological studies consistently suggest lower blood pressures among vegetarians than non-vegetarians independent of age, weight, and pulse rate. Although it is not easy to determine the precise cause of these findings, these studies suggest that some component of animal products, possibly protein or fat, may influence blood pressure in well nourished populations.

As with obesity and hyperlipidaemia, there is evidence of inter-individual variations in susceptibility to hypertension, but the long-term interactions with dietary factors are less easy to discern. Nevertheless the recently collated data from research conducted over decades, shown in Fig. 7 and 8, emphasize the importance of the proposals in previous WHO reports for a primary preventive approach, with interventions geared to limiting the development of obesity and the intake of alcohol and salt. Increased dynamic physical activity may reduce blood pressure independently of its effect on weight change, and an increase in total dietary fat may also have an effect in promoting hypertension as well as obesity. Further research is needed but the evidence for marked environmental effects on blood pressure is clear. A recommendation to maintain normal weight with a diet low in fat and high in complex carbohydrates, and minimize the intake of alcohol is relevant to the avoidance of both obesity and hypertension; a low salt intake may also be beneficial in preventing the rise in blood pressure that is apparent in developed countries from early childhood.

---

[1] Body-mass index = body mass in kg/(height in metres)^2.

3.3 Cancer

The relationships between specific dietary components and cancer are much less well established than those between diet and cardiovascular diseases. This is reflected in reviews of diet and cancer (43–45). However, the overall impact of diet on cancer rates throughout the world appears to be significant. For populations in developed countries, where cancer rates are highest and account for approximately one-quarter of all deaths, some epidemiologists estimate that 30–40% of cancers in men and up to 60% of cancers in women are attributable to diet (*46*).

The evidence for the influence of diet on cancer risk is derived from several sources. Correlations between national and regional food consumption data and cancer rates, and studies of the changing rates of cancer in populations as they migrate from a region or country of one dietary culture to another, have led to many important hypotheses. Case-control studies of the dietary habits of cancer patients and comparison subjects, and prospective studies of populations with known dietary habits, provide stronger evidence for the effects of diet in relation to major cancers. Many of these observations from human populations have been supported by animal experimental data.

Studies of diet in relation to some cancers have been confined to relatively homogeneous populations and have not been replicated across a range of cultural and dietary settings; for other cancers, the research has been pursued over a wider range of dietary intakes. Included among the cancers that have been linked repeatedly to dietary factors in different populations are cancers of the oral cavity, pharynx, larynx, oesophagus, stomach, large bowel, liver, pancreas, lung, breast, endometrium, and prostate.

3.3.1 *Cancers of the oral cavity, pharynx, larynx, and oesophagus*

In developed countries, epidemiological studies clearly indicate that drinking alcoholic beverages is causally related to cancers of the mouth, pharynx, oesophagus, and upper part of the larynx (*47*). There is no indication that the effect is related to the type of beverage. Smoking also causes cancers at these sites. There is also some evidence that cancers of the mouth and throat are increased by poor oral and dental hygiene.

In correlation studies conducted in different parts of the world, investigators have found positive associations between oesophageal cancer and several dietary factors, including (*a*) low intakes of lentils, green vegetables, fresh fruits, animal protein, vitamins A and C, riboflavin, nicotinic acid, magnesium, calcium, zinc, and molybdenum; (*b*) high intakes of pickles, including salt-pickled vegetables, and mouldy foods containing *N*-nitroso compounds; and (*c*) consumption of foods and beverages at very high temperatures. The reported associations are consistent with the general hypothesis that certain nutrient deficiencies, such as are found in many high-risk populations, including heavy alcohol drinkers, might increase the susceptibility of the oesophageal epithelium to neoplastic transformation.

Case-control studies of oral and laryngeal cancers have also shown an increased risk associated with infrequent ingestion of fruit and vegetables.

3.3.2 *Stomach cancer*

A high incidence of stomach cancer is found in Japan and other parts of Asia and in South America, but not in North America or Western Europe where the rates are low and still decreasing. In the United States of America, stomach cancer rates are now among the lowest in the world, whereas in 1930, this was the leading cause of cancer death for men and the second leading cause in women. Gastric cancer incidence is decreasing in Japan, and a gradual decline in incidence over several generations has been noted among Japanese migrants to Hawaii. It seems most likely that these trends are related to changes in food consumption patterns, since several dietary factors have been implicated in gastric cancer risk. Stomach cancer is associated with diets comprising large amounts of smoked and salt-preserved foods (which may contain precursors of nitrosamines) and low levels of fresh fruits and vegetables (acting as possible inhibitors of nitrosamine formation). Dietary shifts away from this pattern could explain the declines in stomach cancer mortality in industrialized nations over the past 50 years, but the evidence is not conclusive.

3.3.3 *Colorectal cancer*

International comparisons indicate that diets low in fibre-containing foods and high in fat increase the risk of colon cancer. The initial suggestion that a lack of dietary fibre might increase the occurrence of large bowel cancer came from observations of the virtual absence of this cancer in southern Africa. The indigenous populations were known to eat a lot of plant foods, and to have much higher faecal weights than populations from industrialized countries.

Several studies also demonstrate positive associations between the risk for colorectal (primarily colon) cancer and dietary fat. In general, the data suggest that saturated rather than unsaturated fatty acids may be responsible for this effect. In other studies, positive associations have been found between meat consumption and this cancer, but many studies have also shown no relationship between fat or meat intake and colorectal cancer. Several case-control and cohort studies provide suggestive but inconclusive evidence that drinking alcoholic beverages, in particular beer, has a causal role in the development of rectal cancer.

The data relating dietary fibre *per se* to colorectal cancer are equivocal. Although several studies have shown inverse relationships between the intake of high-fibre foods and colon cancer risk, these foods (vegetables to a large extent) are rich sources of other nutritive and non-nutritive constituents with potential cancer-inhibiting properties. Lower rates of colorectal cancer in Californian Seventh-Day Adventists, half of whom are vegetarians, support a protective effect of a vegetarian diet, although this group also abstains from alcohol.

In summary, an increased risk of colorectal cancer appears to be associated with high fat intake (particularly saturated fats) and low vegetable intake. It is not clear whether dietary fibre *per se* is protective or whether the apparent effect is due to other food constituents. Rectal cancer risk may be increased by the consumption of beer.

3.3.4 *Liver cancer*

Primary liver cancer is relatively rare in North America and most developed countries, but it is common in sub-Saharan Africa and south-east Asia, where it is associated primarily with exposure to hepatitis B virus infection. Liver cancer incidence and mortality, by geographical area, or among different population groups, have been correlated with aflatoxin contamination of foodstuffs in Africa. On the basis of evidence in developed countries, consumption of alcoholic beverages is causally related to liver cancer (*47*).

3.3.5 *Lung cancer*

In most industrialized countries, lung cancer is the leading cause of cancer deaths among men, and it is rapidly approaching this status among women. The most important causal factor is cigarette smoking. Lung cancer risk in males is clearly increased by certain occupational exposures (e.g., to asbestos, nickel, chromate, or gamma-radiation), several of which have been shown to interact synergistically with smoking.

Studies in several different populations have shown an interactive effect between smoking and a low frequency of intake of green and yellow vegetables rich in beta-carotene. These findings are consistent with experimental data showing tumour inhibition by vitamin A and synthetic analogues. In prospective studies, the frequency of consumption of beta-carotene-containing foods and the concentration of beta-carotene in serum have been inversely associated with the risk of lung cancer, but early reports of a similar inverse association for serum retinol (vitamin A) have not been confirmed in subsequent studies. Dietary fats and dietary cholesterol have also been positively associated with lung cancer risk.

3.3.6 *Female breast cancer*

Several lines of evidence support the importance of dietary factors in the causation of breast cancer. The first derives from animal experimental studies, which have demonstrated that, both with and without the presence of known mammary carcinogens, the incidence of mammary tumours in rats increases substantially with diets high in total and saturated fat, provided that the diet contains a small amount of polyunsaturated fat. A role for fat and other dietary factors is also supported by descriptive epidemiological studies, correlation studies, case-control and cohort studies, and evaluations of nutrition-mediated biological risk factors.

Correlation studies provide evidence of a direct association between breast cancer mortality and the intake of energy, fats, and specific sources of dietary fats, such as milk and beef (see, for example, Fig. 9, page 68). Several case-control studies have associated breast cancer risk with dietary constituents, especially fats. However, not all studies show these relationships.

There is epidemiological evidence—not fully consistent—relating alcohol consumption to the risk of breast cancer in women. It is, at present, unclear whether this association is causal.

3.3.7 *Endometrial cancer*

A strong association between endometrial cancer risk and excess weight has been reported in several studies, and a hormonal mechanism has been postulated for this association. Specific dietary factors other than obesity have not been identified for this disease.

3.3.8 *Prostate cancer*

International incidence and mortality data generally show a positive correlation of prostate cancer with the incidence of other diet-related cancers, including cancers of the breast, corpus uteri, and colon. Inter- and intra-country analyses show positive correlations between mortality from prostate cancer and per caput intake of total fat. These findings have been supported in analytical studies showing an association of prostate cancer with the intake of high-fat foods.

Although studies of certain other cancers suggest that vitamin A and, in particular, beta-carotene may be protective factors, some case-control studies indicate that beta-carotene may be a risk factor for prostate cancer, especially among men aged 70 years and older. Increased weight or obesity has also been positively associated with the risk of prostate cancer.

3.3.9 *Summary and conclusions: major associations between diet and cancer*

Table 11 summarizes the strength of association between dietary components and cancers at various sites. A review of the evidence indicates that a high intake of total fat—and in some case-studies also saturated fat—is associated with an increased risk of cancers of the colon, prostate, and breast. The evidence is strongest for cancer of the colon, and weakest for breast cancer. The epidemiological evidence is not totally consistent, but is generally supported by laboratory data from studies in animals. The experimental data, however, also point to an adverse effect of very high intakes of polyunsaturated fats, at levels that are considerably above current intakes in human populations.

Diets high in plant foods, especially green and yellow vegetables and citrus fruits, are associated with a lower occurrence of cancers of the lung, colon, oesophagus, and stomach. Although the mechanisms underlying these effects are not fully understood, such

Table 11. Associations between selected dietary components and cancer[a]

Site of cancer	Fat	Body weight	Fibre	Fruits and vegetables	Alcohol	Smoked, salted, and pickled foods
Lung				−		
Breast	+	+			+/−	
Colon	+ +		−	−		
Prostate	+ +					
Bladder				−		
Rectum	+			−	+	
Endometrium		+ +				
Oral cavity				−	+ [b]	
Stomach				−		+ +
Cervix				−		
Oesophagus				−	+ + [b]	+

Key: + = Positive association; increased intake with increased cancer.
− = Negative association; increased intake with decreased cancer.
[a] Adapted and extended from reference *44*.
[b] Synergistic with smoking.

diets are usually low in saturated fat and high in starches and fibre and several vitamins and minerals, including beta-carotene and vitamin A. There is no conclusive evidence that these beneficial effects are due to the high fibre content of such foods.

Sustained heavy alcohol consumption appears to be causally linked to cancer of the upper alimentary tract and liver. Excessive body weight is clearly a risk factor for endometrial and postmenopausal breast cancers, but the association of these cancers with excessive energy intake *per se* is less well established.

High fat intake is associated with cancer at several sites. Certainty about the optimum intake of fat in relation to cancer must await future research, such as controlled trials. In the meantime, international correlation analysis (Fig. 9) and other epidemiological data indicate that fat intakes of less than 30% of total energy will be needed to attain a low risk of fat-related cancers. A reduction in risk is also likely when fat intake is reduced towards 30%, especially if this dietary change is combined with a change in other dietary components (Table 11).

In conclusion, although several lines of evidence indicate that dietary factors are important in the causation of cancer at many sites and that dietary modifications may reduce cancer risk, the contribution of diet to total cancer incidence and mortality cannot be quantified on the basis of present knowledge. Nevertheless, evidence indicates that a diet that is low in total and saturated fat, high in plant foods, especially green and yellow vegetables and citrus fruits, and low in alcohol, salt-pickled, smoked, and salt-preserved

Fig. 9. Dietary fat intake in relation to breast cancer-related death rate [a]

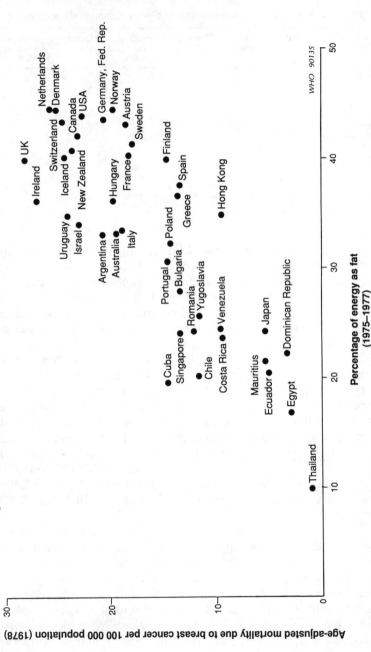

[a] Reproduced from reference 48, by kind permission of the publisher.

foods is consistent with a low risk of many of the current, major cancers, including cancer of the colon, prostate, breast, stomach, lung, and oesophagus.

3.4 Obesity

The occurrence of obesity in individuals reflects the interaction of dietary and other environmental factors with inherited predisposition. However, since there is little evidence that some populations are more susceptible to obesity for genetic reasons, the differences in prevalence of obesity in different populations are largely attributable to "environmental" factors (especially diet and physical activity). Within a single population, those who become obese usually come from overweight families and there is evidence of heritability for obesity. Thus, from a public health point of view, the challenge is to modify the population's environmental circumstances so that the susceptible individual members of the population are less liable to become obese.

3.4.1 Obesity in adults

The state of obesity is normally taken to indicate an excess of body fat, but most analyses of the relationship between body fat and disease have depended on measuring body weight as an index of body fatness. Body weight as a function of height is normally expressed as the body-mass index (BMI):

BMI = body mass in kg/(height in metres)^2.

This expression is useful in adults since it takes account of the increase in weight with increasing height. It is assumed that the same proportions of lean and fat issue are found in people of different height, so that the definition of obesity usually depends on specifying the degree of "excess" weight-for-height. This presupposes an understanding of what constitutes a normal body weight. The definitions are currently based on life insurance statistics, or on long-term epidemiological studies in North America and Europe. There have as yet been no long-term studies to see whether similar grades of excess weight are accompanied by the same risks for those living in developing countries.

There is, however, substantial evidence that in many cultures obese adults develop the same complications, and so the definitions derived from affluent communities should be used universally for the present. A BMI of 20–25 is taken as normal for adults in developed countries (49, 50). If differences in smoking habits are not taken into consideration, then it can appear that moderate overweight is beneficial. Fig. 10 shows, however, that a BMI of 20–25 is appropriate for both smokers and non-smokers. Moderately overweight adults are often non-smokers, whereas among thin adults there is a higher proportion of smokers, who are at a much greater health risk; this distribution produces a U- or J-shaped curve of mortality against weight in the population as a whole. A small increase in risk is also seen below a BMI of 20 in non-smokers, but an appreciable part of this reflects the lower weight of individuals who are already sick.

It should be noted that these BMI values apply to individuals. A population has to have a average value of about 22 to allow almost all the individuals to fall within the 20–25 BMI range. This implies that a substantial proportion of the adult population in developed countries will be classified as overweight since the population average BMIs are often in the range of 24–26.

When dealing with developing countries, it is suggested that the lower limit of "normality" for individuals of 20 is too high and a limit of 18.5 has therefore been proposed on the basis of the usual

Fig. 10. Body weight, smoking, and death rates for men and women[a]

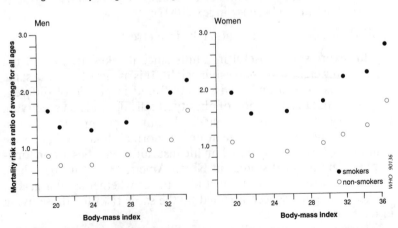

[a] Reproduced from reference 49, by kind permission of the publisher. Recalculated from data in reference 51, with unpublished data from the American Cancer Society.

distribution of adult weights. Although evidence is lacking on the health risks associated with a BMI of 18.5 in developing countries, an average BMI of 20 may be considered appropriate for these countries. Thus, for all countries, a range of average BMIs of 20–22 for the adult population is suggested as acceptable.

Three grades of obesity are also identified (Fig. 11), Grade 1 carrying only moderate health risks but Grade 3 being very severe and carrying high risks of hypertension, coronary heart disease, diabetes mellitus, and gastrointestinal disorders, e.g., gallstones. The risks of cancers of the gallbladder, breast (in postmenopausal women), and uterus are increased in obese females, as are perhaps the risks of prostate and kidney cancer in obese males. Weight is a crude measure of adiposity, but only a few small studies have used more specific measures of body fat. There is increasing evidence, however, that fat deposited abdominally presents a greater hazard, so that a waist-to-hip circumference ratio of more than 0.85 is a particular risk.

4.4.2 Obesity in children

The BMI has not yet been established as a method of assessing obesity in children and adolescents. The present methods for indicating obesity are largely based on defining a weight-for-height in excess of a reference value. Similarly, a weight below a reference

Fig. 11. Degrees of chronic energy deficiency and obesity in relation to body-mass index

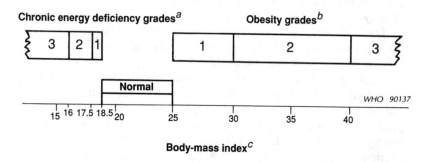

[a] Chronic energy deficiency grades from reference 53. Grades 1 and 2 require that energy expenditure is also below 1.4 times the estimated basal metabolic rate, based on the weight of the individuals.
[b] Obesity grades from reference 52.
[c] Body-mass index = mass in kg/(height in metres)².

71

weight-for-height value is taken as indicative of "wasting". The reference values may be taken as 2 standard deviations above and below the National Center for Health Statistics (USA) standard weight-for-height of children below the age of 11 years (54). For adolescents, the problem is more difficult because children enter their pubertal spurt in growth and rapidly change their body composition and weight during this growth phase. An FAO/WHO/UNU report on energy and protein requirements gives reference standards for adolescents based on data published by Baldwin in 1925 on weight-for-height, in the absence of modern analyses of adolescent weights and body composition in relation to health (55). Further research is needed in this field before definitive reference standards can be set.

3.4.3 *Factors influencing body weight*

Changes in body fat depend on an imbalance between energy intake and energy expenditure. Thus, obesity develops when energy intake is in excess of expenditure for a sustained period of time.

The causes of obesity can be many, but social and environmental factors that either increase energy intake or reduce physical activity place a greater demand on the normal mechanisms of appetite control and metabolic regulation. As societies become more affluent and mechanized, the demand for physical activity declines. This is apparent in many societies and affects both young and old. The fall in physical activity demands that energy intakes should also be reduced if excess energy is not to be stored as excess fat. Therefore, changes in the environment that affect the level of energy expenditure of children and adults may influence the development of obesity.

There is increasing evidence from experimental animal studies, human physiological measures of energy metabolism, and bioenergetic considerations, that dietary fat is particularly conducive to weight gain. Excess dietary fat is more readily stored than dietary carbohydrate, but fibre-rich complex carbohydrates are also much bulkier and tend to limit energy intake. National and international analyses are in keeping with the concept that, as the proportion of energy derived from fat increases. so does the problem of obesity, particularly in susceptible individuals. Thus, in a national household survey in Brazil (see Fig. 12), statistical analyses that took account of a range of factors, including income and the dietary source of typical nutrients, found that the single most important factor

Fig. 12. Household diet and adiposity in Brazil, according to dietary staples [a]

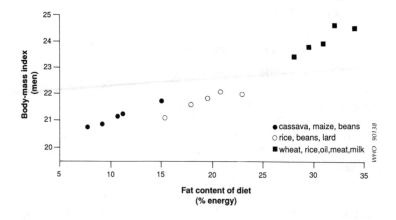

[a] Adapted from reference 56. For each dietary pattern, the households studied were split into five groups according to average annual income, with ranges as follows: ●, US$ 99–418; ○, US$ 220–990; ■, US$ 1700–8500.

associated with different degrees of adiposity in households was the fat content of the diet (56).

The bulkiness of diets low in fat and high in complex carbohydrates is so great that on some African diets children are unable to derive enough dietary energy for their needs, especially when they are unwell with recurrent infections. This has led to the promotion of fat supplementation of infants' and children's diets to ensure adequate energy intakes. A diet with modest amounts of fat, e.g., 15–20% of energy, may avoid problems of energy deficiency without unduly enhancing the hazards of obesity and other chronic diseases that tend to occur in societies with an average dietary fat content above 30% of energy.

Complex metabolic changes occur in individuals who become obese. The treatment of obesity is notoriously difficult because of the prolonged nature of the treatment, the need to readjust dietary energy intakes and/or physical activity permanently to maintain a reduced weight, and the changes in metabolism and in appetite that tend to minimize weight loss. Thus, a preventive policy seems the only long-term solution to the problem of obesity, with a high-risk group within a society being identified as those with a family history of obesity, diabetes, hypertension, or hyperlipidaemia. These individuals have a far greater risk of putting on weight or of developing complications with only modest gains in weight.

3.5 Non-insulin-dependent diabetes mellitus

Non-insulin-dependent diabetes mellitus is a chronic metabolic disorder in which there is impairment of the body's capacity to utilize glucose derived from carbohydrate foods, from body stores of glycogen, or from body and dietary protein. This disease, whose onset usually occurs in middle adulthood, is strongly associated with an increased risk of coronary heart disease (31), with a range of renal, neurological, and ocular disorders, and, during pregnancy, with adverse effects on the fetus.

This type of diabetes is to be distinguished from insulin-dependent diabetes, and from the gestational diabetes of pregnancy. Diabetes may also be associated with malnutrition; fibrocalculous pancreatic diabetes, for example, is found in Latin America, Africa, and Asia.

Obesity is a major risk factor for the occurrence of non-insulin-dependent diabetes, the risk being related to both the duration and the degree of obesity. Approximately 80% of patients with this form of diabetes are obese. The incidence rate of diabetes is almost doubled when moderate overweight is present and can be more than three times as high as normal in the presence of frank obesity.

The occurrence of diabetes within a community appears to be triggered by a number of environmental factors such as sedentary life-style, dietary factors, stress, urbanization, and socioeconomic factors. The prevalence of non-insulin-dependent diabetes mellitus varies from zero in the highland population of Papua New Guinea, which has retained its traditional life-style, to 50% or more in the Pima Indian and Nauruan populations (57).

The most rational and promising approach to preventing non-insulin-dependent diabetes is to prevent obesity. Weight control is of fundamental importance in both the population strategy for the primary prevention of this disorder and the strategy for prevention in high-risk individuals (i.e., persons with impaired glucose tolerance or with a genetic predisposition to diabetes). Physical activity not only improves glucose tolerance by reducing overweight, but also acts independently, by having a beneficial effect on insulin metabolism.

Diets high in plant foods are associated with a lower incidence of diabetes mellitus. In a large follow-up study of Californian Seventh-Day Adventists, the death rate from diabetes mellitus was approximately half that for all whites in the USA (58). Moreover, within that same group, vegetarians had a substantially lower risk than non-vegetarians of having diabetes as an underlying or contributing cause of death. Intervention studies in urbanized Australian Aborigines with impaired glucose tolerance have demonstrated beneficial effects of reversion to a traditional diet.

These observations, and other studies, raise the possibility of the primary prevention of diabetes by dietary means. However, there is as yet insufficient evidence to allow specific dietary goals to be given, other than those for the prevention of obesity.

There is a much clearer scientific basis for the prevention of cardiovascular and other complications in diabetic individuals. Annex 2 summarizes recent recommendations offered by expert groups elsewhere.

3.6 Non-cancer conditions of the large bowel

Certain chronic disorders of the large bowel are thought to occur more frequently in association with the typical "affluent" diet. These include diverticular disease of the colon, haemorrhoids ("piles"), and constipation. Low intake of dietary fibre is considered to be a major cause of these disorders.

3.6.1 Diverticular disease

The relatively hard, concentrated, slow-moving faeces that result from an inadequate intake of dietary fibre are believed to disrupt bowel motility and increase the internal pressure, causing diverticular pouches that can become chronically inflamed, leading to the condition of diverticulitis. In developed countries, this condition is common after the age of 40 years, when it affects an estimated 20% of the population.

3.6.2 Haemorrhoids

When intake of dietary fibre is low, the increased physical effort necessary for defecation may raise the intra-abdominal pressure, thereby increasing pressure in the veins. The surface veins in the lower rectum are considered to be particularly vulnerable to being stretched and weakened by these pressure changes; eventually these veins form dilated haemorrhoids which can become inflamed, or locally thrombose.

3.6.3 *Constipation*

Chronic constipation occurs in about 10% of adults and 20% of the elderly living in societies with low intake of dietary fibre, e.g., a daily intake of about 20 g of fibre, equivalent to about 12 g of non-starch polysaccharides (NSP).[1]

Constipation occurs under controlled feeding conditions when the daily faecal weight falls below about 100 g; in epidemiological studies, faecal weights below 150 g/day are associated with slower transit times of food through the intestine. Above 150 g/day faecal weight, transit times of food through the bowel are little changed.

Fig. 13 shows a well defined linear relationship between NSP intake and mean daily stool weights. From studies conducted on mixed British diets to which cereal fibre was added, an intake of NSP of about 22 g is needed to achieve an average faecal output of 150 g, and to minimize the number of individuals with faecal outputs below 100 g. An intake of 22 g of NSP is higher than the typical intake in European and North American countries. In eastern Finland, however, intakes of 18 g of NSP are observed in populations with no problems of constipation or diverticular disease. This practical figure or intermediate target of 18 g of NSP (or the corresponding figure of 30 g of dietary fibre) has therefore been chosen by European and North American committees when specifying dietary fibre goals.

In rural Africa, daily stool weights are much higher than in developed countries, e.g., 450–550 g/day, and similar values have been observed in rural Malaysia. In Indians on an urbanized diet, and South Americans, faecal weights are also high, e.g., 300–375 g in different age groups. As soon as the diet begins to change towards the European pattern, however, faecal weights fall to 170–300 g/day on average.

Although there is a clear association between NSP intake, stool weight, and constipation, further information is still needed on the

---

[1] These polysaccharides, which contribute to total dietary fibre, are the complex carbohydrate components of the diet other than starches. Since the definition and measurement of dietary fibre *per se* remain uncertain, NSP can be useful as a measurable indicator of fibre intake.

Fig. 13. Mean daily stool output (g) and dietary intake of non-starch polysaccharides in groups of healthy subjects on controlled diets[a]

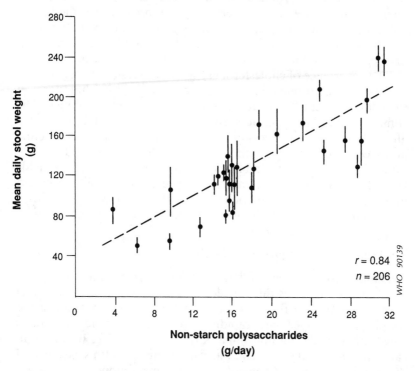

[a] Redrawn from an unpublished paper prepared by J. Cummings for the Department of Health Committee on Medical Aspects of Food Policy, UK.

amounts of NSP eaten in developing countries, and also on the colonic effects of high intakes of starchy foods, some of which (e.g., maize-based porridges and rice) are eaten after cooling. When starches are cooled or refrigerated, a change in their tertiary structure is likely to occur, resulting in an increase in the proportion passing into the colon after ingestion.

3.7 Gallstones

In gallbladder disease, gallstones (predominantly cholesterol gallstones) form within the gallbladder. Gallstones occur much more commonly in developed countries than in developing countries. Within affluent societies, the prevalence is higher in non-vegetarians than in vegetarians. In women, the prevalence increases steadily from around 5% in young adulthood to around 30% in old age; in men, the prevalence rates at every age are approximately one-half of those in women. In symptomatic cases (i.e., approximately one-quarter of all cases), surgical removal of the gallbladder or physical or chemical dissolution of the gallstones is often required.

The occurrence of cholesterol gallstones is a result of the presence of supersaturated bile (i.e., a raised concentration of cholesterol in the bile); this tends to occur more often in women than in men. The composition of bile is particularly affected by dietary factors, and is affected adversely by excess body weight. Overweight adults excrete an excess of cholesterol with the bile, but fibre intake reduces the saturation of cholesterol in bile by altering the recycling of bile acids from the intestine, and the amounts of bile and metabolites excreted in the faeces. A starchy diet rich in fibre may therefore be protective, particularly if it helps to limit the problem of overweight.

3.8 Dental caries, sugars, and fluoride

Dental caries has been a human health problem since antiquity. Until the Middle Ages the prevalence of caries was low. Today, it is a very common health problem affecting a large proportion of people in developed and rapidly developing countries. It causes considerable suffering and impairs the quality of life. In addition, caries places a heavy financial burden on public health services, and the problem cannot be controlled by treatment alone.

Historical surveys have demonstrated that, with the introduction of sugars and refined flour and the manufacture of confectionery and sweet baked foods, caries prevalence increased dramatically over a relatively short period. The prevalence of caries in many developing countries is currently increasing rapidly in response to dietary changes associated with increasing use of products containing sugar. This trend is now in striking contrast to that in the industrialized nations where dental caries has been decreasing in the past 20 years, in response to various preventive measures.

Diet can affect teeth in two ways: first, while the tooth is forming before eruption and, secondly, through a local effect after the tooth has erupted. The post-eruption local effect is much more important, and sugars, in particular sucrose, are the most important dietary factor. Sucrose has greater cariogenic potential than starch; biochemical, microbiological, animal and human clinical, and epidemiological evidence supports a causal relationship between frequent sucrose intake and caries, but many other factors, including individual susceptibility, modify the dental response to sucrose. Glucose alone, or mixed with sucrose and fructose, may also cause caries, so increased emphasis is now being given to the consumption of all free sugars, rather than just sucrose alone, in the development of caries.

Different types of food may increase or decrease caries rates depending on their properties, e.g., stickiness, buffering capacity, or nutrient content. These properties have been intensively investigated by firms that manufacture or sell sugar-containing products in developed countries. Despite suggestions that starch is cariogenic, an extensive review of the evidence (59) showed that cooked staple starch foods such as rice, potatoes, and bread appear to be of low cariogenicity. Fresh fruit, despite its intrinsic sugar content, has a lower cariogenic potential, but the addition of sugar to cooked starchy foods increases the development of caries. Less-refined starchy foods may perhaps, by virtue of their fibre content, help protect teeth from dental caries. Children given carbohydrates as wholemeal bread, beans, oats, rice, potatoes, and fruit with some treacle and molasses develop fewer and smaller carious cavities than do children fed a diet containing the level of sucrose and refined flour typical of an affluent society.

Numerous epidemiological studies conducted at the population level suggest that there is a direct relationship between the quantity and frequency of sucrose consumption and the development of caries. The relationship approximates to a sigmoid (S-shaped) curve that rises more steeply as the consumption of sucrose-containing products increases, after which the curve flattens out, i.e., the increase in dental caries is small with further increases in sucrose intake. In general, very little caries occurs in children when the national consumption level of sugar is below 10 kg per caput per annum, i.e., about 30 g/day, but a steep increase may occur from 15 kg upwards. As a result of rising consumption of sugar and other cariogenic substances in developing countries and the absence of adequate fluoride intake, the prevalence of caries is now higher in some developing countries than in many industrialized countries (7).

The introduction of new sugar-containing products in developing countries, in particular for use between meals, will lead to increased caries incidence, if not immediately met by effective caries-prevention programmes. There is an obvious dilemma—the preventive programmes have to be established first, when the disease level may still be low, and the interest for prevention consequently minimal. Nevertheless, if such programmes are not established while the shift in dietary patterns is still taking place, caries will become a major health problem.

Fluoride has toxic effects on teeth and bone when ingested in excess. Dental fluorosis and skeletal fluorosis are well known effects of fluoride excess. The margin of safety between the range for deficiency and toxicity is narrow. A sufficient daily ingestion of fluoride is needed to prevent dental caries, although there is no consensus regarding the exact amount of fluoride needed (figures of 0.7–1.5 mg of fluoride per day from all sources have been discussed in the scientific literature). In most countries, drinking-water supplies about 75% of daily fluoride intake. Many communities, particularly in temperate climates, have water supplies fluoridated to a level of around 1 mg/litre. Keeping in mind the toxic effects of fluoride, and the high daily intake of water in the tropics, there is a need to prescribe both lower and upper limits in terms of total daily intake. A concentration of 0.6 mg/litre in drinking-water has been proposed for tropical countries. The presence of dental fluorosis within a community is an indication that the total intake of fluoride is too high. Countries with a problem of excess environmental fluoride must try to defluoridate their water supplies. Countries with low water fluoride levels may plan strategies to increase the fluoride intake of the population to the appropriate level by adopting known methods of fluoride supplementation.

3.9 Osteoporosis

As the number of elderly in the population increases, problems of old age can be expected to become a greater burden on health services. Already in the developed world many people die following fracture of the femur, which occurs particularly in older women with fragile bones, after a relatively minor fall. By age 90 years, one-third of the women and one-sixth of the men in the USA will have had hip fractures. In 12–20% of cases, the fracture or its complications will be fatal; half of those who survive will need long-term nursing care (60). Table 12 shows the incidence of hip fracture in different parts of the world. There is a 20-fold range in rates, even when they are adjusted for age. The higher the incidence, in general, the greater the proportion of women affected. In Yugoslavia, inhabitants of the

Table 12. Incidence rates[a] of hip fracture by region and sex[b]

Country, area or population group	Women	Men	Female/male ratio
United States (Rochester, MN)	101.6	50.5	2.01
New Zealand	96.8	35.2	1.79
Sweden	87.2	38.2	2.75
Jerusalem	69.9	42.8	1.63
United Kingdom	63.1	29.3	2.15
Netherlands	51.1	28.5	1.80
Finland	49.9	27.4	1.78
Yugoslavia[c]	39.2	37.9	1.03
Hong Kong	31.3	27.2	1.15
Yugoslavia[d]	17.3	18.2	0.95
Singapore	15.3	26.5	0.58
South African Bantu	5.3	5.6	0.94

[a] Per 100 000 per year, age-adjusted to USA population 1970.
[b] Based on data originally published in: GALLACHER, J.C. ET AL. Clinical orthopedics, 150:163–171 (1980). Reproduced, by kind permission of the publisher, from CUMMINGS, S.R. ET AL. Epidemiology of osteoporosis and osteoporotic fractures. Epidemiologic reviews, 7:178–208 (1985).
[c] Low-calcium diet.
[d] High-calcium diet.

higher-calcium-intake region have a fracture rate half that of those living on the lower-calcium diet. Nevertheless, low rates were observed in Singapore and among the Bantu, where calcium intakes are lower than in the USA. The age-specific rate of hip fracture appears to be rising rapidly for some poorly defined reason, and is now considered to be reaching epidemic levels in many affluent countries (61). Increasing fragility of bone is one major reason for hip fractures, although instability of gait, deteriorating eyesight, and poor neuromuscular reflex coordination also account for the rising incidence of hip fracture with age.

Fragility of bone usually results from osteoporosis in which the amount of bone tissue in a given volume of bone, i.e., the bone density, is reduced. Bone density increases in all parts of the skeleton during childhood and adolescence to reach a peak value at about the age of 20 years and then falls again from the menopause in women and from about age 55 years in men, but at a diminishing rate with advancing age. Women in developed countries lose about 15% of their bone mass in the first 10 years after the menopause, but annual rates of bone loss vary from 0.5% to 2% between individuals. There is a wide range of bone density in healthy young adults, i.e., $\pm 20\%$ of the mean; values below the normal lower limit for the young are defined as osteoporotic. Thus, individuals who reach middle life at the lower end of the normal density range rapidly become osteoporotic with advancing age, whereas those whose mid-life bone density is high may never develop osteoporosis in their natural lifetime. Factors governing the rise in bone density during growth (e.g., genetic, hormonal, nutritional, and exercise) may therefore prove to be very important in determining whether an individual develops osteoporosis.

Known determinants of bone density have been classified under five headings (*61*): (*a*) lack of estrogen, (*b*) immobility, (*c*) smoking, (*d*) alcohol and drug therapy, and (*e*) calcium intake. Estrogen lack in public health terms relates to the decline in estrogen activity in women after the menopause. Bone density is less in people who drink a large amount of alcohol, and their rate of bone loss is greater for reasons that may relate in part to alcohol-induced alterations in hormone metabolism. The traditional emphasis given to calcium intake reflects the recognition of the importance of calcium in contributing to the density of bone during growth and the value of heavy, initially dense, bones in adult life. Calcium supplements may also be helpful in reducing the rate of bone loss in postmenopausal women, but at levels of intake that are pharmacological rather than nutritionally relevant. It is by no means certain that calcium intake is the key feature determining bone density and bone loss in adult life. High-protein and high-salt diets, for example, are known to increase bone loss.

Fracture risk is a continuous inverse function of bone density; the age-related decline in bone density (together with the increased incidence of falls) produces the age-related rise in fracture incidence that is a feature of all human societies. Women are more prone to these fractures than men because their peak bone density is lower, they suffer accelerated bone loss after the menopause, and they live longer than men. Populations in developing countries appear to be less at risk from fracture than those in developed countries, despite their lower body weights and calcium intakes, possibly because they smoke less, drink less alcohol, do more physical work (which promotes bone formation), and consume less protein and salt (both of which increase obligatory calcium loss from the body).

Little is known of the factors underlying the variation in osteoporosis around the world. Studies in developing countries are few but dietary trends that diminish calcium intakes or increase protein and alcohol intakes may have adverse effects on bone density. A decline in physical activity and an increase in smoking rates are also likely to increase the risk of osteoporosis, and these two factors may explain the currently increasing problem of hip fractures in the developed world, where widespread smoking has occurred for about 50 years, i.e., during the adulthood of many women and men who are now falling victim to hip fractures.

Recent studies from India clearly show that osteoporosis occurs in population groups subsisting on low-calcium traditional vegetarian diets and living in areas where the drinking-water contains high concentrations of natural fluorides. Similar observations have been made in China and the United Republic of Tanzania. Unlike the osteoporosis of the geriatric population in affluent societies, this type of osteoporosis in the developing countries affects cortical bones throughout the body, and is found in a younger age group. The significant feature, however, is that the combination of a diet low in calcium and a high fluoride intake causes metabolic bone disease characterized by osteoporosis; where dietary levels of calcium are high, no osteoporosis is found despite a high intake of fluoride.

3.10 Chronic liver and brain diseases, and other effects of alcohol

Alcohol consumption has many adverse health effects, many of which are strongly associated with the age of exposure and with the amount consumed. In middle and older age, alcohol consumption influences the risks of a range of chronic disease processes, particularly of the liver and brain.

Liver cirrhosis is the major chronic disease caused by alcohol consumption (62). The liver's capacity to metabolize alcohol is surpassed when consumption is excessive; toxicity results and liver cells are destroyed, to be replaced by scar tissue. In developed countries, at least 40% of fatal liver damage is due to alcohol. There is evidence that women are more susceptible to this cirrhogenic effect of alcohol than are men. Long-term excessive consumption of alcohol has a variety of other adverse effects on the gastrointestinal tract and pancreas (47).

Another important chronic effect of alcohol consumption is brain damage, entailing mood disorder with confabulation (Korsakoff's syndrome) or a state of delirium and cranial nerve palsies (Wernicke's encephalopathy). It takes about 10 years of heavy drinking to produce these brain damage syndromes; alcohol appears to accelerate aging processes that interfere with the capacity to reason and solve the problems of everyday living.

Alcohol consumption influences the occurrence of coronary heart disease and hypertension (see also section 3.2). While people who consume low-to-moderate amounts of alcohol are at a slightly lower risk of coronary heart disease than are abstainers, many epidemiological studies have shown that moderate or heavy consumption of alcohol is associated with increased blood pressure, and abstinence from alcohol is followed by a fall in blood pressure. Hypertension contributes to an increased risk of coronary heart disease and stroke.

As discussed in section 3.3, alcohol is a causal factor in various cancers, including cancers of the liver, larynx, mouth, throat, and oesophagus, and, perhaps, cancer of the rectum and, in women, cancer of the breast (47).

Alcohol also causes serious health problems at younger ages. There is a characteristic pattern of abnormalities, recognized over the past two decades, in newborn babies of mothers who drink alcohol heavily during pregnancy (63). This "fetal alcohol syndrome" involves general retardation of growth, including mental retardation, a characteristic "flat" face with small eyes, lowered bridge of the nose and lack of normal folds, and other anomalies such as congenital heart disease. The fully developed form of the syndrome occurs predominantly in the children of women consuming more than eight alcoholic drinks per day. However, other effects on the fetus, such as low birth weight and an increased risk of stillbirth, occur at levels of intake greater than two drinks (or 20 g of alcohol) per day. Estimates from North America and Europe indicate an incidence of fetal alcohol syndrome of 1–3 per 1000 live births and of some adverse effects in a further 3–5 per 1000 live births. Alcohol is therefore one of the most common causes of birth abnormalities in developed countries.

In adults, particularly young adults, the importance of alcohol in motoring accidents is well established. In developed countries, between one-third and one-half of deaths on the road have alcohol as a significant causal factor. Alcohol is also a major factor in other accidents such as drownings and boating accidents, and in industrial accidents and absenteeism.

3.11 Food contaminants, food additives, plant toxicants, marine biotoxins, and mycotoxins in relation to chronic diseases

Various non-bacterial contaminants of foods cause "acute" diseases, often in epidemic form but sometimes in sporadic form.

These noncommunicable diseases can affect the liver and nervous and skeletal systems and are associated with a high case-fatality rate.

3.11.1 *Food contaminants*

Residues of pesticides and veterinary drugs

Since 1963, FAO/WHO joint meetings have been held regularly to consider pesticide residues in food. Limits have been recommended by the Codex Alimentarius Commission for residues of pesticides and herbicides permitted in agricultural produce, and practical limits for the levels of these residues in the environment have been established for approximately 120 compounds. The number of Codex limits for specified foods now exceeds 3000. In establishing the limits, careful attention is given to good agricultural practice, and the pesticides are evaluated toxicologically for their safety in food. These toxicological analyses include animal testing and studies of the metabolism of the chemicals in humans; groups of workers exposed to higher amounts of these chemicals are also monitored to ensure that there is no evidence of harm. The Codex limits assume that these chemicals are properly used.

However, if the chemicals are improperly used, without rigorous control and monitoring, serious harm may result. Few data are available on the long-term health effects of the misuse of these chemicals, although animal data suggest the possibility of a profound long-term impact on health.

Residues resulting from the application of drugs in animal husbandry and veterinary medicine have been under review by the Joint FAO/WHO Expert Committee on Food Additives for several years. Codex-recommended limits have been established, giving careful attention to good husbandry practice. No evidence of harm to humans has been found when approved drugs are used and Codex-established limits are not exceeded.

Heavy metals

Serious chronic diseases have been reported when foods containing large quantities of cadmium, lead, or mercury have been ingested over extended periods of time. Continuous surveillance is needed to ensure the safety of the food supply.

Other environmental contaminants

Evidence of disease caused by other environmental chemicals such as polychlorinated biphenyls and dioxins is rare. This may be due to large-scale underreporting, to the great difficulty in correlating exposure with the possibly latent effects, or to the fact that these chemicals occur generally only in minute amounts in food.

3.11.2 *Plant toxicants*

Toxicants in edible plants and poisonous plants resembling them (mushrooms, certain wild green plants) are important causes of ill-health in many areas of the world. In some places, the poorer sections of the population eat plants known to be potentially toxic (e.g., *Lathyrus sativus*) in order to combat hunger. Pyrrolidizine alkaloids are frequent contaminants of edible millet, and cause liver diseases. Contamination of edible oil can cause epidemic dropsy and has been linked to other epidemics.

3.11.3 *Marine biotoxins*

A WHO Expert Committee convened in cooperation with FAO in 1973 considered fish and shellfish hygiene (*64*), including the principal diseases resulting from the ingestion of, or contact with, fish and shellfish, the principal diseases of these animals, the biotoxins of marine fish and shellfish, the surveillance and epidemiological investigation of fish- and shellfish-borne diseases, and the safe handling of fish and shellfish and their products; in addition to the Committee's report (*64*), two books on these subjects have been published by WHO (*65, 66*).

Surveillance of foodborne disease due to fish and marine biotoxins is grossly inadequate in many regions of the world, especially in developing countries, in which the number of such outbreaks is not known with any accuracy.

3.11.4 *Mycotoxins*

At least 150 different types of mould, when growing on certain foods under suitable conditions, produce substances (mycotoxins) that are toxic to humans or animals (*67*). Because of the formation of mycotoxins, the general problem of mould growth on foods has extensive agricultural and economic implications beyond obvious food spoilage. This has been of particular importance when developing programmes for growing protein-rich foods based in part on peanuts, cottonseed, soya, and other plant sources, for use in the alleviation of malnutrition.

The most extensively studied mycotoxins, e.g., aflatoxins, are generally resistant to normal food-processing techniques. Some mycotoxins are powerful carcinogenic agents in animals and probably also in humans; others cause ergotism, alimentary toxic aleukia, and other diseases.

The control of mycotoxicoses requires that mould contamination in food and animal feed should be prevented or reduced to harmless levels. This demands good agricultural practice in harvesting, drying, handling, storage, transportation, and distribution procedures (*68*).

3.11.5 *Food additives*

Food additives are used for four main purposes:

—to preserve the nutritional quality of foods;
—to maintain the safety of food by inhibiting the growth of bacteria or other organisms that might cause serious illness;
—to improve the consistency of foods, for example to make them thicker or easier to spread;
—to make food look more attractive in colour and to improve the taste.

Since 1956, food additives have been under continuous toxicological evaluation by the Joint FAO/WHO Expert Committee on Food Additives. The Codex Alimentarius Commission has established maximum permitted limits for the safe use in foods of evaluated additives. Specifications for the identify and purity of food additives have also been published by FAO and WHO to ensure that only those of food-grade quality are used. The effects of additives on health are under continuous review to ensure that they do not lead to ill-health in the amounts recommended by the Codex Alimentarius Commission. There is, however, the risk that the illegal use of chemicals in food can mask poor quality, disguise food deterioration, or constitute a deliberate adulteration of the product. The adulteration of food can, in certain circumstances, be very harmful to health besides damaging the consumer's perception of the identity and value of food.

Some traditional food additives (e.g., curing salts, smoke) are considered to be risk factors for certain diseases, for example for hypertension and some cancers. Their use should be carefully monitored or, where possible, they should be replaced by other preservation methods proved to be safe. Rules for the safe preparation of food for immediate consumption have been published by WHO (see Annex 3).

4. INTEGRATING INFORMATION ON NUTRITIONAL AND DIETARY RELATIONSHIPS TO DISEASE

4.1 Nutrients

Section 3 summarized the relationship of some aspects of the diet to the development of specific chronic diseases. Many national and international committees have considered in detail the causes of cardiovascular diseases, cancers, and other conditions of public health importance. However, it is essential to integrate the conclusions if a coherent public health policy is to be developed.

In theory, it is possible for a specified intake of a nutrient to increase the risk of one disease while decreasing the risk of some other disease; further, this relationship could itself vary for different segments of the population. The policies for preventing those two diseases could therefore be very different, and could lead to a complicated set of policies linked to different subsections of the population. Fortunately, this problem does not seem to arise, since the dietary recommendations for preventing most of the conditions prevalent in developed countries are very similar (see section 3). It is still necessary, however, to consider the optimum intake of specific nutrients needed to prevent each condition, and whether any inconsistencies occur.

It is also important to assess the relationship of particular foods or diets, rather than nutrients, to certain diseases since there may be insufficient evidence to identify the specific nutrients responsible for the effects of particular diets. Given the remarkable variety of dietary habits in different countries, it would also be helpful to know which of several different diets are compatible with long-term health. This section therefore attempts to integrate current knowledge about different components of the diet; it also deals in some detail with diets high in plant foods and with alcohol intake.

4.1.1 Dietary energy

The energy utilization of an individual is finely controlled by physiological mechanisms, and adjusts to changes in the individual's size and pattern of physical activity. Deliberate decreases in energy intake lead to progressive changes in body weight, to additional small adaptive metabolic changes amounting to about 10% of total energy expenditure, and perhaps to alterations in physical activity. The reproductive performance of women appears to be impaired by insufficient energy intake, and a child's growth will be slowed or stopped and spontaneous physical activity restricted when food intake is inadequate. If food is freely available, then food is consumed in response to the demands of the body; the larger the individual and the more physically active, the greater the energy need. However, the metabolic flexibility of the body is limited, and it is difficult to introduce major changes in energy intake for more than a few days before hunger or satiety signals will tend to limit further weight changes. Changes in the energy density of foods, such as brought about by introducing sucrose- and/or fat-rich foods low in complex carbohydrates and fibre, will produce effects that will become apparent over a period of weeks or months. The cumulative effect of a sustained 2% discrepancy between energy intake and energy expenditure can lead in an adult to a 5 kg weight change over a period of one year. Thus, consideration of the selective effects of different sources of energy in promoting overweight and obesity is important in public health terms.

The energy intake of populations varies substantially, but this does not necessarily reflect differences in energy requirements. A recent analysis of per caput energy requirements of different populations conducted for FAO has assessed the importance of a variety of factors in determining the energy needs of different populations (69). In developing countries, the population is predominantly young with therefore a lower average energy requirement and the adults are also usually shorter with a lower body weight. Although physically more active, particularly in rural areas, men and women in developing countries usually have a lower energy requirement than North Americans simply because their body weight is lower.

The smaller body size reflects an earlier constraint on physical growth and development. In addition, physical activity itself, although at a relatively high level, may be restricted as an adaptation to insufficient energy intakes (55). Thus, as populations of developing countries gain access to unlimited food and benefit from improved conditions of water and food hygiene, and as the prevalence of infectious diseases declines, they may be expected to grow taller and possibly to become more active. The future food needs of such countries will therefore increase even if the population does not increase. Population growth remains, however, the dominant factor determining projected food needs.

Once the overriding need for food energy to meet the requirements for children's growth and adults' economic and social activities has been met, then the effects of different sources of energy can be considered. Protein requirements are readily met in children and adults eating a varied diet based predominantly on cereals and pulses, and these diets, which are consumed by the majority of the world's population, provide on average about 10–15% of the total energy from protein. There are no known advantages from increasing the proportion of energy derived from protein, and high intakes may have harmful effects in promoting excessive losses of body calcium and perhaps in accelerating an age-related decline in renal function.

On average, 85–90% of dietary energy will be derived from non-protein sources, i.e. from carbohydrate, fat, and alcohol. The arguments presented in this report discourage the use of alcohol as an energy source and encourage a limitation on fat intake. The lower limit on fat intake is based upon consideration of both essential fatty acid requirements and of energy density. In practice, diets low in total fat are seen most frequently in developing countries. In that setting, the diets tend to be high in "bulky" foods and concern exists that the total volume of food may restrict energy intake in young children and the elderly. The Study Group concurs with an earlier assessment of this situation (70) and proposes that the lower limit for the average fat intake by a population group be set at 15% of dietary energy. At this level of intake, needs for essential fatty acids can readily be met and the problems associated with the bulk of food can be handled. Appreciably higher fat intakes may nevertheless be needed by infants and very young children, and particularly in countries where food practices must allow catch-up growth of children with various degrees of malnutrition.

4.1.2 *Fat consumption*

As the total fat content of the diet increases, an increasing proportion of persons within the population—including, particularly, the most susceptible individuals within that population—develop obesity with all its complications, e.g., diabetes and hypertension. Studies on the control of energy balance in humans have not yet shown differences between saturated and unsaturated fatty acids, so the total amount of fat seems to be the important consideration in the prevention of obesity. There are no good systematic studies on the prevalence of obesity in relation to the proportion of fat in a nation's diet, but crude analyses of the national food supply (from FAO figures) in relation to the average body-mass index, measured as part of the recent major Intersalt study on adults, suggest that a mean body-mass index of 22–23 is associated with a dietary fat content that provides 15–20% of energy (*11*). In Brazil, the mean BMI is about 22 and the fat content of the diet amounts to 18% of energy intake, on average. Fig. 3 (page 30) shows that in Brazil the prevalence rate of obesity is low in children. European figures suggest that, for adults, a mean BMI of 25–26 is associated with a dietary fat content that provides 35–40% of energy. There is then a prevalence of Grade 1 obesity of about 40% in middle-aged men and women. On the grounds of obesity alone, therefore, any increase in fat intake beyond perhaps 20% of energy should be avoided.

Table 11 (page 67), which summarizes the links between diet and cancer, suggests that a high intake of total fat may also promote the development of a number of cancers. The evidence cannot be considered sufficiently strong to be termed causal, but most expert groups now consider it prudent to reduce fat intakes in Western societies from the prevailing figure of about 40% of energy towards the 20–30% figure (see Annex 4).

Total fat intake has also to be considered in relation to cardiovascular disease. The level of total fat intake does not affect blood cholesterol concentration unless appreciable amounts of saturated fat are consumed. Fat intake as such may, however, promote the development of hypertension. Total fat intake, therefore, needs to be restricted on this basis. Again, a figure of 30% of energy or less has been suggested as acceptable and this value is also advocated in the management of diabetes mellitus, where the risk of cardiovascular complications is very high (see Annex 2).

One further reason for specifying a population mean intake of total fat within the range of 15–30% of energy for the prevention of cardiovascular disease is the need to restrict saturated fatty acid intake. Most diets in developed countries contain an excess of saturated fatty acids, so policies that lead to a fall in total fat intake are also likely to reduce the diet's saturated fat content.

Thus, there is a coherence in the prevention policies dealing with all these conditions. It is therefore possible to identify an upper limit for fat intake of 30% of energy for the population average. However practical considerations in some developed countries suggest that it would be sensible to have an intermediate shorter-term target of 35% as the upper limit, to allow the changes in the food and agriculture industries to occur progressively without any major disruption caused by extreme and abrupt changes in policies. These difficulties emphasize, however, the importance that developing countries should attach to arresting uncontrolled increases in the fat content of their diets (see section 6).

4.1.3 Intakes of saturated fatty acids

Saturated fatty acids and cholesterol are not essential nutrients and their importance relates directly to their effects in increasing blood cholesterol concentrations and promoting the development of coronary heart disease. As noted previously (section 3), no lower limit to serum cholesterol has been identified below which a beneficial reduction in coronary heart disease cannot be expected (Fig. 14) so national nutrition policies should seek to minimize intake of saturated fatty acids. These fatty acids may also be specifically involved in promoting cancers, particularly of the colon and breast, although the evidence remains inconsistent. The main justification for limiting saturated fatty acid intake should therefore be the prevention of coronary heart disease.

Adults in rural areas of developing countries where they have particularly low blood cholesterol concentrations, of 3.24–3.89 mmol/l (125–150 mg/dl), eat a diet with a saturated fatty acid intake of 3–5% of energy and a total fatty acid intake of 5–10% of energy; these intakes represent the practicable minimum for such regions. The WHO Expert Committee on the Prevention of Coronary Heart Disease (*31*) advocated a limit of 10% of energy to be derived from saturated fatty acids. Recent evidence reinforces the validity of this recommendation, but northern European committees have taken a

Fig. 14. Serum cholesterol level and incidence of new coronary heart disease (any type) in different populations and subgroups [a]

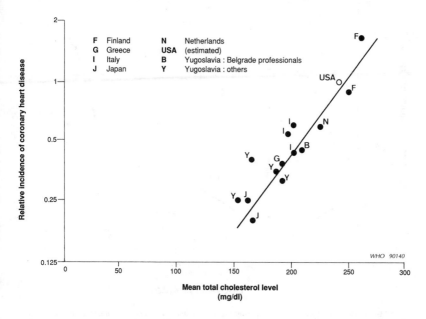

[a] Calculated from reference 30, adapted by R. Peto, and redrawn with permission.

pragmatic intermediate goal of 15%, while advocating a more rigorous change of diet to bring saturated fatty acid intakes below 10% in individuals at high risk, e.g., those who are overweight, hypertensive, or hyperlipidaemic. Since the increase in mortality (predominantly from coronary heart disease) is progressive throughout the body-weight range (Fig. 15) (49), and since the same is true for blood pressure (Fig. 7, page 59) and blood cholesterol concentrations (Fig. 14), the definition of high-risk groups within a population is necessarily somewhat arbitrary and based on the relationship of the group to the average for the population—which may itself be considered at high risk. Thus the choice of intermediate nutrient goals is a policy decision based on issues other than health, e.g., economic or social considerations.

Dietary cholesterol also has a significant impact on blood cholesterol concentrations, but its effect is less than that of changes in intake of saturated fatty acids. A policy of limiting cholesterol

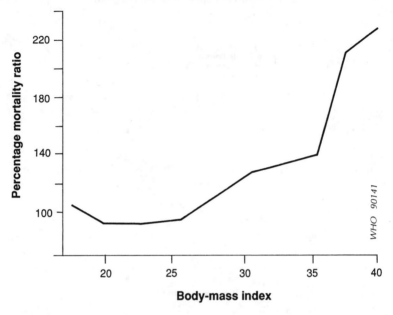

Fig. 15. Mortality in relation to body weight for men aged 15–39 years[a]

[a] Redrawn from reference 49, by kind permission of the publisher. Data recalculated from the Build Study. Men were followed up for 22 years. Mortality is expressed as a percentage of the average for the entire group.

intake to less than 300 mg/day seems to have almost universal agreement.

4.1.4 Total carbohydrates

In all diets, total carbohydrate intake consists mainly of complex carbohydrates, the remainder being made up of free or unrefined sugars.

The basis for specifying a national target for intakes of free sugars of 15–20 kg per person per year, provided that fluoride intake is sufficient, has been set out previously (74). This intake amounts to 40–55 g of free sugars daily, which corresponds to about 6–10% of the daily energy intake. Other reasons for limiting intakes of free sugars have been cited, including concerns about the development of obesity and, thereby, diabetes and cardiovascular disease, but there is little evidence that sucrose or other free sugars have specific effects

94

that would warrant a lower intake than that recommended to minimize the problem of dental caries.

Any greater intake, however, could be disadvantageous in that free sugars in the diet displace other energy sources such as starches which, when obtained from cereals, pulses, and vegetables, are accompanied by a wide variety of micronutrients. It therefore seems appropriate to obtain 50–70% of energy from complex carbohydrates derived from these sources. Given the widespread concern about vitamin and mineral deficiencies over the last 50 years, it would be unwise to prejudice the nutritional gains obtained by improving the nutrients available in the diet by the addition of a nutrient-free source of energy. Similar arguments can apply to the increase in dietary energy from fat which provides only a few nutrients, e.g., fat-soluble vitamins. Alcohol is also an important energy source which is often accompanied by few if any nutrients. Thus, sucrose, fat, and alcohol are all capable of displacing other energy sources of nutritional quality because appetite is primarily geared to the control of energy intake.

As the proportion of the elderly increases in a population, the issue of the nutrient density of the diet will also become more important because energy requirements fall progressively in the elderly, although their needs for protein, calcium, iron, and other nutrients either remain the same or actually increase. Thus, the nutritional quality of the diet needs to change in old age, i.e., at an age when people usually seem to maintain their traditional patterns of eating. A policy of maintaining a high quality diet throughout life therefore seems appropriate; both sucrose and other free sugars and, to a lesser extent, fat should therefore be limited on nutritional quality grounds alone. Given a suggested intake of 50–70% of energy from complex carbohydrates, an upper limit of 10% of energy from free sugars would appear to be the maximum if an appropriate 10–15% of dietary energy is to be derived from protein and 15–30% from fat.

4.1.5 Complex carbohydrates

The relationships seem to be consistent between the levels of complex carbohydrate in the diet and the risks of the various diseases reviewed in section 3. The proposals that 50–70% of energy should come from complex carbohydrates are based on a variety of considerations that do not necessarily relate to the nutritional qualities of these food components as such. They relate mainly to the recognition that diets rich in complex carbohydrates are useful in preventing excessive weight gain, limiting hyperlipidaemia, and managing diabetes, and seem to favour a lower incidence of a variety of cancers.

Nutritional research into the positive benefits of complex carbohydrates as such is limited, but the benefits from the minerals and vitamins associated with them are many. Many of the plant sources of complex carbohydrates provide, for example, the essential fatty acids, rich sources of calcium, zinc, and iron, and a variety of water-soluble vitamins. Complex carbohydrates can affect colonic function as well as the normal absorptive mechanisms in a variety of ways that may contribute, by as-yet-unknown mechanisms, to their many nutritional benefits.

4.1.6 *Cereal intakes*

Cereals provide the principal source of starch in most communities, and the arguments in favour of a substantial cereal intake are widely cited, as noted in section 3. Cereals also provide a rich source of dietary fibre; cereal fibre is particularly resistant to bacterial degradation in the colon and thereby contributes to faecal bulking and the avoidance of constipation. For adults, the suggested minimum average intake of non-starch polysaccharides (NSP) is 22 g/day (see section 3 for background). This proposal is based exclusively on the need to avoid constipation and the associated problems found in affluent societies with low fibre intakes. A high starch intake also contributes to faecal bulking, because resistant starch, as well as normal undigested starch, enters the colon to provide a substrate for colonic metabolism.

As yet, too little is known about the relative advantages of high-starch diets with a moderate rather than a high fibre content, so the suggested NSP target of 22 g/day may change in the light of new research. This figure of 22 g of NSP corresponds to a value of about 37 g of total dietary fibre, measured by the older enzyme methods of the 1970s, which is consistent with the figure suggested for the management of diabetes or of individuals at high risk of coronary heart disease in North America or Europe. Therefore, a figure of 22 g of NSP, or 37 g of total dietary fibre, is suggested as a target for the present, this fibre to be derived predominantly from cereal and vegetable sources. It should be recognized, however, that the second figure of 37 g depends greatly on the type of diet consumed in a country, because different sources of food give different values for total fibre by the rather unreliable older methods. The analysis of NSP is more consistent, but there is as yet no international agreement on fibre measurement techniques.

For adults, an upper recommended average of 32 g of NSP can be suggested from the progressive increase in faecal output as NSP intake rises (Fig. 13, page 77). Other data suggest that, above an intake of 32 g of NSP, the response in faecal output is less predictable, and that this high intake is more than adequate to ensure that the whole adult population is prevented from having constipation. A daily intake of 32 g of NSP should therefore represent an upper limit. The lower limit is specified as 22 g/day to reduce the likelihood of adults having a faecal output below 100 g/day.

The relationship illustrated in Fig. 13 was derived from studies of European and North American adults. Account of the lower food intakes of children, and of adults of smaller size and stature, must therefore be taken in deriving population averages. Values have been derived by taking the average energy requirements for countries with many children and adults of short stature, to ensure that too high a value is not chosen in absolute terms. This approach leads to lower and upper average limits for the whole population of about 16 g and 24 g of NSP.

To simplify the handling of the fibre data, the information can also be expressed in rounded figures as a proportion of energy. Thus, the average lower and upper limits for NSP are 2.2 g/MJ and 3.2 g/MJ, respectively (9 g/1000 $kcal_{th}$ and 13 g/1000 $kcal_{th}$). In terms of total dietary fibre, the corresponding figures are about 3.7 g/MJ and 5.3 g/MJ (15 g/1000 $kcal_{th}$ and 22 g/1000 $kcal_{th}$). These values allow the more ready application of the recommended limits to distinct population groups of different age structures.

One potential source of concern with fibre-rich diets is whether their phytate or oxalate content will limit the availability of minerals such as calcium, zinc, and iron. Studies from the eastern Mediterranean region suggest that very high intakes of unleavened bread, where the cereal phytate has not been destroyed by the endogenous phytase of the grain, do lead to problems of mineral malabsorption. However, this seems to be a problem of food preparation rather than of the diet as such. In human physiological studies, exchanging full grain cereals for refined starches low in fibre does not lead to calcium, zinc, or iron malabsorption, because the whole grain provides an additional intake of the minerals that compensates for any reduced mineral availability. Oxalate-rich foods such as spinach do, however, limit mineral absorption. The intake of fibre from a mixed diet providing the maximum proposed adult limit of 32 g of NSP has been shown to allow the maintenance of mineral balance, but this conclusion may not apply to fibre-rich foods made by the addition of bran, which contains extra phytates as well as fibre.

Further research in the field is needed, but for the present the lower and upper population goals of 16 and 24 g of NSP per head per day seem appropriate.

4.1.7 *Intakes of vegetables, fruit, and pulses*

Vegetables and fruits are a rich source of a number of nutrients. They are relatively low in energy but high in fibre, vitamins, and minerals. Thus they form a useful component, contributing to the balance of the diet. In addition, although no precise dose–response relationships between intakes and disease have been reported, there seems to be some consistency in the evidence that vegetables and fruits play some protective role in preventing the development of cancers (see Table 11, page 67). It is not known whether their effects on cancer development are nutritionally based, e.g., attributable to the provision of vitamins E and C and beta-carotene involved in free-radical scavenging, or whether other components of these foods exert powerful effects.

Available information (*1*) indicates that, in 1979–81, vegetables and fruits together, globally, provided about 4.5% of energy supply. This figure is believed to be an underestimate because of the consumption of non-marketed vegetables and fruit in many countries. This amount of energy would correspond to about 200 g of vegetables or fruit per day per person. Pulses, nuts, and seeds were estimated to contribute 2.4% of the energy in developed countries and 5.6% in developing ones.

With a view to providing a balanced and sufficient intake, China has recently adopted a national goal of 400 g per day of vegetables and fruits. On the basis of observed national intakes for regions or countries, e.g., southern Italy and Greece, where high intakes are associated with low rates of coronary heart disease and of some types of cancers, a per caput intake of 400 g/day of vegetables and fruits (potatoes, other tubers, and cassava not included) is considered desirable, and of this 30 g/day should be pulses, nuts, and seeds. Potatoes, roots, and other tubers are also a rich source of nutrients in many countries where they may substitute for cereals.

4.1.8 *Salt*

On a population level, the habitual level of salt intake is strongly related to normal blood pressure. In populations with a salt intake of less than 3 g/day, no rise in blood pressure with age was observed, in contrast to populations with a salt intake of more than 6 g/day. Salt may also play a role in the causation of stomach cancer. Therefore an average salt intake of less than 6 g/day is recommended.

4.2 Potential health consequences of diets high in plant foods

The nutrient goals recommended in Table 13 (see page 108) translate into a diet that is low in fat (especially in saturated fat) and high in carbohydrate (especially in complex carbohydrate). Such a diet would be characterized by frequent consumption of vegetables, fruits, cereals, and legumes, rather than by substantial intakes of whole-milk dairy foods, fatty meats, and free sugars. A substantial amount of epidemiological and clinical data indicates that a high intake of plant foods and complex carbohydrates is associated with a reduced risk of several chronic diseases, especially coronary heart disease, certain cancers, hypertension, and diabetes (see section 3).

Although some of this evidence is derived from observational studies of religious groups such as Seventh-Day Adventists, who may differ from the general population in more than just their dietary practices, much of the evidence comes from epidemiological studies, or from controlled trials. Overall, the evidence indicates that diets high in plant foods entail lower risks of various chronic diseases than the current diets of affluent communities.

The possibility of adverse consequences from consuming diets high in plant foods must also be considered. For example, at the population level the consumption of starchy foods is correlated with a higher risk of stomach cancer, and a positive association between starchy foods and stomach cancer has been reported in several, but not in all, epidemiological studies. This positive association is probably attributable to the frequent consumption of salted, pickled, and smoked foods, which tends to accompany a high consumption of starchy foods. Overall, the evidence indicates that diets high in plant foods, and low in salted, smoked, and pickled foods, are associated with a low risk of several cancers, including stomach cancer.

The iron obtained from vegetarian diets may be all in the inorganic form, if no animal foods are consumed; such iron is less well absorbed than iron from non-vegetarian diets, which includes haem iron in meat. However, the absorption of inorganic iron is enhanced by the simultaneous consumption of vitamin C, which is abundant in most plant foods. In North America, iron deficiency anaemia appears to be no more prevalent among vegetarian women than among non-vegetarian women.

The type of diet high in plant food that might be derived on the basis of the proposed nutrient goals—and that may contain foods of animal origin—should be distinguished from the various vegetarian diets prevalent in certain developing and even some developed countries. It is not possible to evaluate the health benefits of diets high in plant foods from studies in developing countries. "Vegetarianism", or a primary reliance on foods of plant origin, is prevalent in many forms in developing countries, especially in India, but the macronutrient composition (or the distribution of food groups) in these vegetarian diets may differ from diets based on the nutrient goals proposed here. For example, diets of low-income Indians are often cereal-based and low in fat and sugar, but they are also often devoid of vegetables and fruit and deficient in various nutrients. Alternatively, the more affluent urban populations in India often consume a fruit- and milk-based vegetarian diet which, while relatively low in saturated fat, is increasingly high in total fat, sugar, and salt. Although the heavily cereal- and fruit-based diet of the urban middle class in India might be expected to entail a low risk of chronic diseases, there are no relevant epidemiological data available.

The risk of deficiencies of protein and of other nutrients may increase as the number of different foods included in individual diets decreases. Diversity in the availability and use of foods must therefore be a key component of any programme aimed at maintaining or improving nutritional health. The role of foods of animal origin is dealt with in section 2.

4.3 Alcohol

Excessive alcohol consumption increases the risk of hypertension (and stroke), liver cirrhosis, alcoholic brain damage, and various cancers. Although there is some evidence that beneficial effects may occur at low levels of alcohol consumption (around 10–20 g of alcohol per day), including some reduction in risks of coronary heart disease and of cholesterol gallstone formation, this remains uncertain.

The higher the average alcohol consumption within a population, the more frequent the associated health problems become. However, because of the very skewed distribution of alcohol consumption, it is not possible to specify an average population level of alcohol consumption that is acceptable from a public health point of view. In many developed countries, alcohol consumption is a long-established and entrenched social behaviour. The public health challenge in these countries is to reduce the average level of consumption among drinkers to a low level (e.g., to around 4% of total energy intake), *and* to eliminate alcohol abuse and high-risk behaviour (especially drinking alcohol in association with driving a motor vehicle). In countries where alcohol consumption is not an established social behaviour or is not acceptable, it is desirable that abstinence be maintained.

4.4 Importance of physical activity

The energy expended in physical activity may be conveniently described in quantitative terms as the proportion of energy expended in excess of the total amount needed to maintain bodily function under basal conditions (basal metabolic rate) and to provide for normal growth, pregnancy, and lactation, and for the energy cost of ingesting and processing food (dietary-induced thermogenesis). The component needed for physical activity often constitutes no more than 20–30% of the total energy expenditure under everyday living conditions. This amount of dietary energy should be enough to maintain physical fitness and to allow for a variety of economically necessary and socially desirable activities.

During the process of development, communities often evolve, from rural societies where physical activity is needed for agricultural production, to more industrialized, urbanized, and affluent societies where the demand for physical labour becomes progressively less. Sedentary activities under these conditions become a more

101

prominent feature. Given the intrinsic advantages of physical activity (see below), it is unfortunate that the decrease in the demand for physical work during normal occupational activity is not counterbalanced by a substantial increase in leisure-time activity. There is, therefore, a progressive decline in total energy expenditure from physical activity as societies become more affluent and industrialized.

Inactivity and a sedentary life-style have several adverse consequences for health. Research now clearly indicates that several physiological functions associated with health may be compromised by a decline in physical exertion. A summary of the body functions affected by the decline in physical activity is set out in Fig. 16, which also enumerates the multiple benefits of regular exercise.

Special attention should be paid to the maintenance of appropriately high levels of physical activity at earlier ages, as many diet-related disturbances (e.g., obesity) develop during childhood and adolescence. Daily activity patterns at these ages are being increasingly influenced by very sedentary leisure-time activities, such as watching television or the playing of electronic games for several hours per day.

It is not possible to differentiate clearly between the benefits of short periods of intense exercise and the benefits that accrue from prolonged periods of modest activity and which are, on a 24-hour basis, of a similar energetic significance. It appears that the effects of prolonged periods of moderate activity, such as occur among populations in developing countries, are as beneficial as the physiological changes that occur in response to the episodic bouts of vigorous exercise characteristic of sporting, leisure-time activity in affluent societies. On this basis, it seems reasonable to conclude that the maintenance of reasonable levels of physical activity on a daily basis should be the principal concern of societies where mechanization and leisure-time activities are conducive to a sedentary life-style. (In order to maintain cardiovascular "fitness", it has been suggested that aerobic activity sustained for periods of at least 20 minutes, three to five times per week at a level of between 50% and 85% of the maximum oxygen uptake capacity, is appropriate.)

Various clinical trials and epidemiological studies have established the association of regular physical training with improved glucose tolerance and reduced insulin levels. Physical activity also increases the concentration of circulating high-density

Fig. 16. Physiological functions and capacities that improve
with regular exercise (left) and the various diseases and conditions
that are influenced favourably by these changes (right) [a]

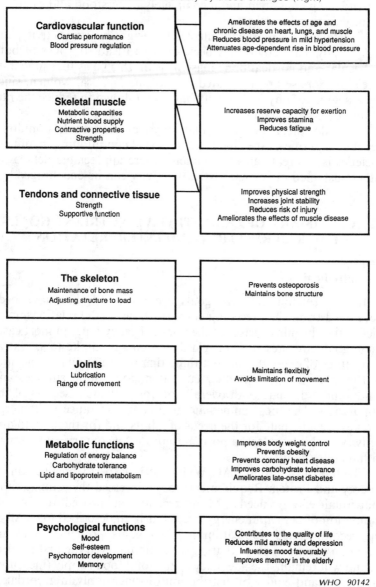

[a] Adapted with permission from reference 71.

lipoprotein cholesterol and tends to reduce systolic and diastolic blood pressure. The relationships between cancer and physical activity are inconsistent and incompletely understood and therefore require further investigation.

Skeletal mass is markedly affected by weight-bearing activity, and lack of physical activity has been shown to lead to a loss of both trabecular and cortical bone mass. It is on this basis that moderate levels of exercise are advocated for postmenopausal women, since these degrees of physical activity have been shown to reduce the rate of loss of bone calcium.

It would therefore seem that physical activity has multiple benefits, and one of the challenges of social conditioning in affluent societies is to create an environment where appreciable degrees of either sustained or intense physical activity can be encouraged.

5. A SUMMARY OF QUANTITATIVE NUTRIENT GOALS, THEIR DERIVATION AND INTERPRETATION

5.1 Introduction

In this section, nutrient goals are presented that have been developed from the preceding considerations of the relationship of diet to the chronic diseases of the non-deficiency type. In most cases these goals are presented in relation to energy intake (e. g., fat as percentage of energy). The first thing that most national authorities will wish to know is whether current national food supplies and intakes are adequate both overall and for individual sectors of the population. The most immediate goal is an assurance that energy intakes are adequate for the needs of adults and for the growth and activity of children. It is important to protect a country's investment in human capital.

The report of a joint FAO/WHO/UNU Expert Consultation on Energy and Protein Requirements (55) addressed the estimation of individual energy needs. More recently, a procedure for the estimation of per caput energy needs has been described (69). All of the recommended population nutrient goals presented here are based on the assumption that, at the national level, the first priority is, and will remain, the adequacy of the total food supply (measured as energy) and equity of distribution of that supply in accordance with individual needs.

Section 2 of this report addresses some of the diseases of nutritional inadequacy now common in certain population groups of most countries of the world, including both protein–energy malnutrition and specific nutrient deficiencies. An early task in any given country will be to ensure that the food supplies and intake patterns are adequate to prevent deficiencies in both macronutrients and micronutrients. This must be a high priority for most developing countries, where nutritional deficiencies are a continuing problem (*4*). Nothing in the present report should be seen as reducing that first priority.

The particular focus of the present report is on the non-deficiency chronic disease states resulting from dietary imbalances. These diseases have attracted more attention in the industrialized countries than in the developing countries. Nevertheless, it is clear that the same chronic diseases are emerging as important concerns in the developing countries—for the more privileged sectors at present, but for the whole population in the future.

The population nutrient goals proposed in this report are designed to address the situation in which the total intake of energy is reasonably appropriate, but where the balance of macronutrients (protein, fat, carbohydrate) is inappropriate and is a major contributing cause of chronic disease. The goals proposed are appropriate for developed and developing countries alike. This report should be seen as complementary to, not a replacement for, earlier FAO/WHO reports on nutrient requirements (and on food and nutrition planning—see list of references), and to previous WHO reports on chronic diseases that identify other risk factors and approaches to their control.

5.2 Concepts

It is the specific recommendation of the Study Group that population approaches to the control of chronic diseases should be introduced as a part of nutrition policy in all countries. The report has been prepared with this goal in mind. The definition of population nutrient goals is based upon this concept. Since a population approach to the definition of goals may differ from the approaches seen in many other nutrition reports, and will differ also from the individualized approach of curative medicine, the following paragraphs present a conceptual overview.

The fundamental focus of the population approach is the population as an entity. It is assumed that certain problems require an approach that considers the population as a whole, if the health problems of individuals within that population are to be addressed effectively (72).

Most nutritional reports have addressed the estimated needs of individuals and have attempted to identify the minimum intake that would meet the nutritional needs of essentially all individuals. Recent reports have taken cognizance of the fact that excessively high intakes of essential nutrients may have detrimental effects (6, 55). The concept of a safe range of intakes, sufficiently high to avoid dietary inadequacies and sufficiently low to avoid detrimental effects of excess, has evolved. The present report follows that lead, but focuses upon the maintenance of low population risk rather than low individual risk.

The approach of this report is to identify the level of population intakes that, for the population as a whole, will lead to a low risk of inadequacy and a low risk of excess. It is the entire distribution of intakes, characterized by the average per caput intake, that is of interest, not the intakes of particular individuals. The concept is illustrated in Fig. 17. (See Annex 5 for discussion of relationship of this concept to that of the "recommended intake" or "safe level of intake" applied to individuals.)

The **population nutrient goal** represents the population average intake that is judged to be consistent with maintenance of health in a population. Health in the population is, in this context, marked by a low prevalence of diet-related diseases in the population.

Seldom is there a single best value for such a goal. Instead, consistent with the concept of a safe range of nutrient intakes for individuals (55), there is often a range of population averages that would be consistent with the maintenance of health. If existing population averages fall outside this range, or trends in intake suggest that the population average will move outside the range, health concerns are likely to arise. Sometimes there is no lower limit. This implies that there is no evidence that the nutrient is required in the diet and hence low intakes should not give rise to concern.

The **population nutrient goals** recommended for use in all parts of the world are presented in Table 13. They are expressed in numerical terms, rather than as increases or decreases in intakes of specific

106

Fig. 17. Concept of a population nutrient goal [a]

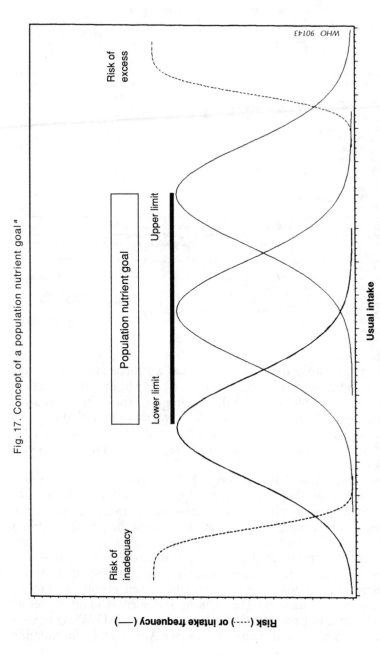

Usual intake

[a] The frequency distributions of nutrient intakes of three hypothetical populations are indicated by the three bell-shaped curves. The risks associated with inadequacy and excess are shown at the two extremes. Populations with mean population nutrient intakes in the range between the lower and upper limits avoid significant risks of inadequacy and excess (prepared by G. Beaton; see also references 6, 55).

107

Table 13. Population nutrient goals

	Limits for population average intakes	
	Lower	Upper
Total energy	see important footnote [a]	
Total fat (% total energy)	15	30 [b]
Saturated fatty acids (% total energy)	0	10
Polyunsaturated fatty acids (% total energy)	3	7
Dietary cholesterol (mg/day)	0	300
Total carbohydrate (% total energy)	55	75
Complex carbohydrate [c] (% total energy)	50	70
Dietary fibre [d] (g/day)		
As non-starch polysaccharides (NSP)	16	24
As total dietary fibre	27	40
Free sugars [e] (% total energy)	0	10
Protein (% total energy)	10	15
Salt (g/day)	– [f]	6

[a] Energy intake needs to be sufficient to allow for normal childhood growth, for the needs of pregnancy and lactation, and for work and desirable physical activities, and to maintain appropriate body reserves of energy in children and adults. Adult populations on average should have a body-mass index (BMI) of 20–22 (BMI = body mass in kg/[height in metres]^2).

[b] An interim goal for nations with high fat intakes; further benefits would be expected by reducing fat intake towards 15% of total energy.

[c] A daily minimum intake of 400 g of vegetables and fruits, including at least 30 g of pulses, nuts, and seeds, should contribute to this component.

[d] Dietary fibre includes the non-starch polysaccharides (NSP), the goals for which are based on NSP obtained from mixed food sources. Since the definition and measurement of dietary fibre remain uncertain, the goals for total dietary fibre have been estimated from the NSP values.

[e] These sugars include monosaccharides, disaccharides, and other short-chain sugars produced by refining carbohydrates.

[f] Not defined.

nutrients, because the desirable change will depend upon existing intakes in the particular population, and could be in either direction. Thus, for example, in some developing countries, the population nutrient goal for fat intake (lower limit) might suggest that it would be desirable to increase average intakes slightly. Conversely, for most of the industrialized countries, a reduction in fat intake is seen as desirable.

In Table 13, and in the body of the report, major attention is directed towards the energy-supplying macronutrients. This must not be taken to imply a lack of concern for the other nutrients; rather, it is a recognition of the fact that, except for protein, previous FAO and WHO reports have provided limited guidance on the meaning of a "balanced diet" described in terms of the proportions of the various energy sources, and that there is now an apparent consensus on this aspect of diet in relation to effects on the chronic, non-deficiency diseases. The present statement should therefore complement, not replace, the existing series of FAO/WHO reports on energy and nutrient requirements (see Annex 1). In formulating policy, requirements for micronutrients as well as the population nutrient goals must be taken into account.

5.3 Derivation of population nutrient goals

In the following paragraphs, a concise summary of the rationale underlying the derivation of population nutrient goals is provided. Previous sections have illustrated the evidence of the relationship of these nutrients to health.

TOTAL FAT	Lower limit 15% of energy
	Upper limit 30% of energy (interim goal)

The evidence is clear that the risk of certain types of cancer is directly associated with the level of total fat in the diet. At present, the range over which the relationship holds is not clear. It may extend across a range of total fat intakes from > 40% of energy down to 20% or lower. There is suggestive evidence that obesity may be associated with high total fat intake, but again there is no specific lower level that marks the end of the relationship.

The Study Group specifically advocates a high intake of complex carbohydrates. As noted below, in terms of energy intake, fat, protein, and carbohydrate together add up to 100%. Since the recommended range for protein intakes is relatively narrow, it follows that the higher the goal set for fat, the lower must be the goal for complex carbohydrates. The Group judged that for the present an upper limit of the population nutrient goal should be set at 30% on the basis of the above considerations. Such a level is consistent with the recommendation offered below that the intake of saturated fatty acids should not exceed 10% of energy. The Group recognized that as additional, more definitive evidence accumulates for cancer, it may be necessary to lower the upper limit for total fat intake to 20–25% of energy.

The health concern associated with low levels of fat in the diet relates to the energy density of diets and the total bulk of food that has to be consumed if energy needs are to be met. This is of greater concern for some developing countries, where diets are based heavily upon cereals and other foods low of energy density, and for the diets of young children and the elderly in whom the volume of food may limit its consumption. The Group supported the conclusion of an

FAO/WHO expert consultation (*36*) and recommended that the lower limit of total fat intake be set at 15% of energy intake. This level of intake would be adequate to provide for essential fatty acid needs.

SATURATED FATTY ACIDS	Lower limit 0% of energy Upper limit 10% of energy

As noted in section 3.2, epidemiological data suggest that as intake of saturated fatty acids decreases there is a progressive fall in mortality due to cardiovascular disease. However, for populations with average intakes below about 10% of energy, there is little additional fall. The Study Group accepted 10% as the upper limit of the range of the population nutrient goals for saturated fatty acids. Since there is no known requirement for saturated fatty acids *per se* (except as a part of the total intake), the lower limit has been set at 0% of energy.

POLYUNSATURATED FATTY ACIDS	Lower limit 3% of energy Upper limit 7% of energy

Polyunsaturated fatty acids include the essential fatty acids required for human health. There is an absolute requirement for their inclusion in the diet. From a review of evidence currently available, the Study Group concluded that diets that provided at least 3% of energy as polyunsaturated fatty acids would be adequate to meet these needs. There have been suggestions that diets with excessively high levels of polyunsaturated fatty acids may be detrimental to health. While this evidence remains uncertain, there is no known advantage to high levels. The Group noted that existing population average intakes seldom exceeded 7% of energy as polyunsaturated fatty acids, even when total fat intake was relatively high. It chose to identify the upper limit of the population nutrient goal as 7% of energy, as a caution against any future rise to very high levels of intake of these fatty acids. When considering polyunsaturated fatty acids, the Group specifically dissociated its recommendations from any notion of a desirable ratio of polyunsaturated fatty acids to saturated fatty acids (P : S ratio), noting that past emphasis on that ratio, rather than on a reduction in intake of saturated fatty acids, may have promoted a progressive increase in the consumption of polyunsaturated fatty acids in some populations.

The Group offered no specific recommendations on the intake of mono-unsaturated fatty acids, noting only that this class of fatty acids would make up the difference between the total fat intake and the sum of the saturated and polyunsaturated fatty acids.

TOTAL PROTEIN	Lower limit 10% of energy
	Upper limit 15% of energy

The lower and upper limits for total protein were set as a reflection of the existing range of average protein intakes in populations around the world in developing and developed countries. The Study Group found no evidence that existing protein intakes are either inadequate or excessive provided that energy needs are being met, that a reasonable range of protein sources (usually both vegetable and animal) is included in the diet, and that due attention is paid to the control of infectious diseases in children (see discussion in section 2.1).

TOTAL CARBOHYDRATE	Lower limit 55% of energy
	Upper limit 75% of energy

The foregoing recommendations account for 25–45% of the total energy intake as fat and protein. Since the Group does not recommend that alcohol be ingested, it follows that the remaining energy intake will be provided by carbohydrate, for which the lower and upper limits for the population nutrient goals are therefore set at 55% and 75%. The Group saw specific advantages associated with the intake of complex carbohydrates and has proposed a lower limit for this class (50% of energy). It was concerned also about excessive intake of sucrose and other free sugars. While goals have been expressed as percentage of energy, it is noted that the goals for protein, fat, and carbohydrate components may not add to 100% with all combinations of upper and lower limits. The Group therefore emphasized that the intent is to maximize the intake of complex carbohydrates and minimize the intake of free sugars, while holding food sugars, notably lactose from milk, to levels consistent with the appropriate usage of the food sources.

COMPLEX CARBOHYDRATES	Lower limit 50% of energy Upper limit 70% of energy

The Study Group noted increasing evidence of specific beneficial effects of complex carbohydrates on intestinal function, on the chemistry of the gut and the physiology of the gut wall with a possible relationship to cancer, and on the absorption and metabolism of carbohydrates and other energy sources (including short-chain fatty acids formed by fermentation in the lower intestine) in relation to the amelioration of diabetes and other metabolic diseases. At present, the available evidence does not lead to the definition of specific population nutrient goals. Rather, it argues in favour of maximizing the intake of this class of carbohydrate, taking into account the energy provided by fat and protein. The lower and upper limits were set on that basis.

DIETARY FIBRE (expressed as non-starch polysaccharides)	Lower limit 16 g/day Upper limit 24 g/day

The population nutrient goals for dietary fibre have been established on the basis of direct experimental evidence concerning the association between dietary fibre and stool bulking (and intestinal transit time), i. e., on the basis of intestinal function. The lower and upper population nutrient goals for NSP may also be expressed as 2.2 and 3.2 g/MJ. The 16 and 24 g levels of NSP are consistent with estimates of about 27 and 40 g of total fibre, which includes other fibre components.

FRUITS AND VEGETABLES	Lower limit 400 g/day
PULSES, NUTS, AND SEEDS	Lower limit 30 g/day (as part of the 400 g of fruit and vegetables)

For the purpose of this recommendation, "fruits and vegetables" does not include potatoes, other tubers, or cassava. The recommendation is made recognizing: the epidemiological evidence of an increased risk of cancer with low intakes of certain fruits and vegetables; the continuing problems of vitamin A deficiency and low availability of dietary iron, which would be ameliorated with increased intakes of vitamin A (or beta-carotene) and ascorbic acid, respectively; and the specific contribution that these groups of foods make to micronutrient and protein intakes. The population nutrient goals have been set judgementally rather than on the basis of specific evidence as to the necessary level of intake. The recommended lower limit is higher than current intake in many populations and much higher than current intake in some of the developed countries. No upper limit has been suggested. The carbohydrate, lipid, and protein contributions of the fruits and vegetables are included within, not in addition to, the previously stated goals.

| FREE SUGARS | Lower limit 0% of energy |
| | Upper limit 10% of energy |

Dental caries rates increase progressively with increases in population sucrose intake. However, the relationship is confounded since oral hygiene practices (including the use of fluoridated toothpastes), the detergent and scrubbing effects of the particular foods eaten, and the frequency of ingestion of sucrose all affect its role in dental plaque formation and dental caries. Thus, the effect is influenced by the life-style of the particular population. It now also appears that other commonly used sugar-based sweeteners have cariogenic effects generally comparable to those of sucrose. The other concern relating to excessive use of free sugars is that they provide energy without associated nutrients and hence displace nutrient-containing foods. For all of these reasons the Group judges that the upper limit of the population nutrient goal for free sugars should be about 10% of energy. There is no lower limit.

| SALT | Upper limit 6 g/day |
| | Lower limit not defined |

The basis of the recommendation for salt intake lies in the association between sodium intake and hypertension, particularly

113

among populations with mean salt intakes above 6 g/day. Since sodium is an essential element, it is clear that there is a lower limit to the population nutrient goals. However, it is not necessary to specify a lower limit for population mean intake. The existing population mean intakes appear to exceed whatever may be the actual limit. Although sodium is the important component, the goal is expressed in terms of salt (sodium chloride). It refers to total sodium chloride intake (all sources) and not just to salt added to foods.

| DIETARY CHOLESTEROL | Upper limit 300 mg/day |
| | Lower limit   0 mg/day |

The Study Group noted that there is evidence that serum cholesterol levels respond to dietary cholesterol intakes. The effect is weaker than that seen with saturated fatty acid intake. There is also epidemiological evidence that mortality due to coronary heart disease is related to dietary cholesterol intake even when the analyses are controlled for serum cholesterol level. High dietary cholesterol intake may therefore convey a risk in its own right, over and above any effect upon serum cholesterol levels. While accepting this evidence as an indication of detrimental effects associated with a high intake of cholesterol, the Group did not find a clear basis for setting a specific upper limit for dietary cholesterol. A consensus of views suggests an upper limit of 300 mg/day. Since there is no requirement for dietary cholesterol, the lower limit is zero. A reduction in intake of saturated fatty acids would be expected also to reduce the intake of fat from animal sources, and hence of cholesterol.

ENERGY INTAKE

The main recommendation of the Study Group was that energy intakes be adequate to maintain desirable levels of body weight (see page 69), to support normal pregnancy and lactation, as well as normal growth rates in children, and to permit required work and participation in leisure activities. The concepts underlying this recommendation have been presented elsewhere (55). Since per caput energy needs vary with a number of characteristics of the population, it is not appropriate to specify quantitative population nutrient goals for energy. The estimation of per caput energy needs has recently been dealt with in detail (*69*).

5.4 Comparison of population nutrient goals with other dietary recommendations

In the past decade, a large number of expert groups associated with government agencies or with voluntary health organizations have issued statements on dietary goals, or recommendations aimed at maintaining good health or preventing specified chronic diseases (usually cardiovascular diseases or cancer). While most recommendations have been directed towards the population, in some cases these same goals, or variations thereof, have been proposed for individuals identified or considered to be at high risk for specific diseases. In most of the statements issued, no clear distinction has been made between goals for a population mean intake (as specified in this report, Table 13) and guidelines intended for individuals. Annex 4 summarizes the recommendations issued in more than 20 countries and regions of the world.

A comparison of the tables in Annex 4 suggests that there are very few major differences in dietary recommendations in different countries, despite the differences in the stated objectives (for maintenance of general health or prevention of specific diseases), in target populations, and in the composition of the committees involved. Sometimes a comparison of such recommendations may make them appear more consistent than is really the case because there may be a tendency for one group to adopt the recommendations of another. Conversely, such a comparison allows consideration of whether groups focusing upon maintenance of general health (Table A4.1), heart disease (Table A4.2), or cancer (Table A4.3) have moved towards consistent advice (Tables in Annex 4, pages 180–185). Experts continue to differ in their judgement about the relative roles of diet and other environmental factors in the causation of specific chronic diseases, and hence about the potential impact of dietary modification on disease risk. Nevertheless, the types of modification recommended by different groups are, in general, similar.

Table 14 compares the population nutrient goals proposed in the present report with recommendations summarized in Tables A4.1–A4.3. For the purpose of this comparison, it has been assumed

115

Table 14. Comparison of the Study Group's recommended population nutrient goals with published recommendations

Nutrient	Study Group's population nutrient goal		National upper or lower limit recommendation[a]		
	Lower limit	Upper limit	Lowest	Highest	Median
Total fat (% energy)	15	30	15	35	<30
SFA (% energy)	0	10	8	15	<10
PUFA (% energy)	3	7	10	13	10
P:S ratio[b]	–	–	0.45	1.2	1.0
Cholesterol (mg/day)	0	300	225	300	<300
Total CHO (% energy)[c]	55	75	40	70	55
Complex CHO (% energy)	50	70	–	–	–
Dietary fibre (g/day)					
As NSP	16	24	–	–	–
As total dietary fibre	27	40	20	35	30
Free sugars[d] (% energy)	0	10	9	25	<10
Salt (g/day)	–[e]	6	5	10	7

SFA, saturated fatty acids; PUFA, polyunsaturated fatty acids; P:S, ratio of polyunsaturated to saturated fatty acids; CHO, carbohydrate; NSP, non-starch polysaccharides.

[a] Values for total fat, SFA, cholesterol, sugar, and salt are upper limits (the median value therefore implies that total fat intake, for example, should be less than 30% of energy); other nutrient values are lower limits (the median value therefore implies that PUFA intake, for example, should be greater than 10% of energy).

[b] Earlier reports specified P:S ratios. Later reports offered recommendations on classes of fatty acids but not on ratios. In this report, care is taken not to specify a ratio, because the SFA value could in theory be reduced to 0%, but the Study Group recommends that PUFA intake should remain between 3% and 7%.

[c] Most reports suggest that most of the carbohydrate should be complex carbohydrate without specifying a specific proportion.

[d] These sugars include monosaccharides, disaccharides, and other short-chain sugars produced by refining carbohydrates.

[e] Not defined.

that the published recommendations referred to population means, unless the original report explicitly stated otherwise. As noted above, many did not specify the exact intent.

The important message from Table 14, and from the more detailed information in the annexes, is that a clear consensus has emerged. The most notable difference is that the upper limit for polyunsaturated fatty acids proposed in this report is lower than that generally recommended. This reflects both the actual upper range of reported population intakes, and concern about the possible effects of excessive intake. The lack of distinction between population-based and individual-based recommendations may also partly explain the difference. For example, the only report that makes separate recommendations for individuals and for populations (45) proposes a population mean intake of polyunsaturated fatty acids of about 7% of energy and an individual intake target of less than 10%.

Unlike most national groups, dealing with only one population, the Study Group recommends both upper and lower limits for nutrient intakes in recognition of the fact that some populations have intakes below the range, and would be advised to increase them towards the minimum, while others have intakes above the maximum and would be advised to reduce them. At a national level, only one direction of change would be applicable. The other refinement of the present report is the specification of lower and upper limits of intake for complex carbohydrate. Previous reports have offered comparable recommendations for intake of total carbohydrate and have suggested that it should be largely in the form of complex carbohydrate, including dietary fibre. If differences in the manner of describing dietary fibre (as non-starch polysaccharides or total dietary fibre) are taken into account, the recommendations are comparable.

The present report does not include specific estimates of energy requirements in the tabulated recommendations, and it does not include recommendations on alcohol intake, although both are frequently included in national reports. These topics were, however, discussed by the Study Group, and the final recommendations made are consistent with those offered previously.

In conclusion, even though not all expert groups have prepared quantitative recommendations, addressed all of the nutrients or all of the disease states, or adequately distinguished between population goals and individual goals, there seems to be a clear consensus on the desired directions of change, and even on the quantitative goals where they have been specified. There do not appear to be major differences between the dietary goals developed within industrialized and developing countries even though, so far, only a few developing countries have published specific dietary goals relating to the prevention of chronic diseases (other than deficiency diseases).

5.5 Population goals versus individual goals

It was noted above that many reports have been ambiguous about the intended application of the goals or guidelines presented. In the present report the Study Group is explicit in emphasizing that the population nutrient goals refer to population averages. If they were applied to the diets of individuals (each individual being urged to meet the population goal), the aggregate change would be substantially greater than is intended by the Group. The phenomenon is illustrated in Fig. 18.

Fig. 18. Distinction between a population nutrient goal and an individual nutrient goal [a]

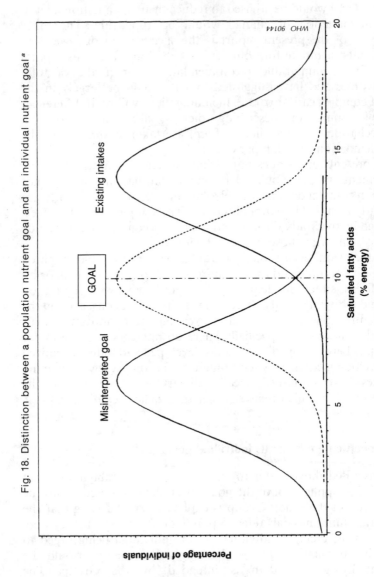

[a] This figure depicts the distribution of intakes of saturated fatty acids for three hypothetical populations, corresponding to: an existing population whose intake is higher than recommended by the Study Group (right); a population that has achieved the *population goal* of a maximum intake of 10% of energy as saturated fatty acids (centre); and a population in which nearly all individuals have an intake less than 10%, a situation that represents the result of misinterpretation of the population goal as an *individual goal* (left) (prepared by G. Beaton).

Those involved in formulating guidelines for individuals, for application in national programmes, might wish to consider the approach used by the US National Research Council committee (*45*) outlined in full in its report. That committee developed both individual and population goals that were compatible with each other and took into account the expected variation in individual intakes around a population mean.

5.6 Population approach versus high-risk individual approach

Over the past 20 years, there has been considerable disagreement about the best approach to the prevention and control of cardiovascular disease. Specifically, it was recognized that serum cholesterol was a measure of risk of coronary heart disease in the individual. Through screening or other programmes, it was possible to select individuals at very high risk and enter them into individually adjusted and individually monitored intervention programmes of a dietary and/or pharmacological nature. Many held that this was the appropriate approach to the control of cardiovascular disease.

The present Study Group does not consider that this approach is an effective way of controlling a problem that is manifest in the population as a whole. There are several cogent arguments for this view, as presented below.

First, although serum cholesterol is a documented predictor of individual risk, this predictor is effective only for those at very high risk. That is, for individuals with serum cholesterol levels in the range seen in the majority of the population, it does not discriminate well between the individuals who will and will not develop coronary heart disease. However, most of the deaths from coronary heart disease occur among this group (see Fig. 19). There are two implications of this observation. If individual interventions are directed only to the high-risk group, at best a small proportion of all the deaths from cardiovascular disease will be delayed or averted. Conversely, if the screening criteria are adjusted to select for intervention in the subpopulation in which events will occur, a very high proportion of the total population will have to be selected. Health care systems, even in the most prosperous of countries, cannot afford such a broad base of individualized intervention. On these grounds, it must be concluded that the individualized high-risk approach will be ineffective in controlling cardiovascular disease

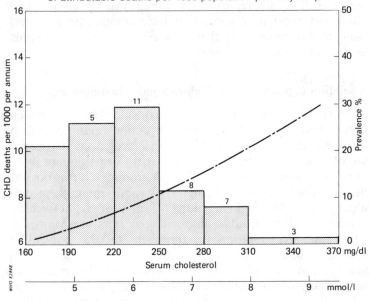

Fig. 19. Prevalence distribution (histogram) of serum-cholesterol concentrations related to coronary heart disease mortality (interrupted line) in men aged 55–64 years. The number above each column represents an estimate of attributable deaths per 1000 population per 10-year period[a]

[a]Adapted from reference 73.

mortality unless a much better indicator of risk than serum cholesterol becomes available.

Second, for cancer there are, at present, no diet-related markers of individual risk that are even comparable with serum cholesterol. There is therefore no possibility of an individualized high-risk approach. Only population interventions are feasible. (For obvious risk factors such as smoking, however, an individualized approach, accompanied by population-based health promotion, is effective for both cardiovascular disease and cancer.)

Finally, and perhaps most important, if the objective is primary prevention, then one must see the whole population as potentially at risk and countries must act before markers of individual risk, such as serum cholesterol, reach levels that would warrant "high-risk intervention". Such markers are secondary to the development of the underlying condition that precipitates clinical disease. When populations are compared, as in the Seven Country Study, the clear conclusion is reached that, in most developed countries, the population is "sick" and the population must be treated (72). The high mortality rates are symptoms of the population illness. This message has particular importance for the developing countries, since the early signs of the population illness are already becoming apparent. They have an opportunity to practise "primordial" prevention at a population level, i. e., to ensure that the population never changes its life-style to one where risk factors are evident. The industrialized countries, or most of them, face the task of, at best, practising primary prevention, by attempting to change life-styles to reduce the pre-existing range of risk factors. Often this has to be combined with secondary prevention for those who already have the clinical disease.

None of the foregoing suggests that individual screening and intervention should not be undertaken. Such an approach is effective for high-risk individuals, but because it is very demanding of resources, it can never be an effective way, by itself, of controlling the problems that now exist in the populations of many developed countries. It is recognized also that, within populations, it may be possible to identify sectors at greater risk and, if resources permit, to direct special programmes towards these sectors. However, such approaches must not be allowed to draw attention away from the fact that the population as a whole may be at relatively high risk and that population-based interventions may be warranted.

6. NUTRITION AND FOOD POLICIES: PAST EXPERIENCE AND IMPLICATIONS FOR ACTION

6.1 Introduction

A distinction should be made between specific policies relating to nutrition, food production, or food security and a food and nutrition policy in which all the objectives of policies for food and for nutrition are integrated. The immediate goal of a *nutrition policy* is the integration of nutrition objectives into different sectoral strategies of national and international organizations. The policies relate directly to the specific nutrient intakes of the populations as a whole, and of subsections of those populations. The immediate goal of a *food-production policy* is to make food available to meet the demands of the population, as well as to provide foreign exchange. At the household level, *food security* aims to guarantee all families access to their minimum food requirements, and this implies that both the availability of foods and the purchasing capacity of the population must be assured. A food policy that relates only to the provision of foods does not incorporate a nutritional perspective.

The Study Group stressed the need to integrate food production with a nutritional objective. This does not deny the immense contributions that an increased availability of food has made to improving the well-being of children and adults, particularly in the developing world. This improvement is manifest by a decline in the number of wasted and poorly growing children and underweight adults. These outcomes have also been partly the result of major sustained efforts to improve water supplies and sanitation, and to provide the education that is often a vital component of the marked improvements in human welfare achieved in developing countries.

The objective of preventing chronic disease has, however, introduced a new urgency to the need to link the wider range of demands in a nutritional policy with food-production policies. In addition to making food available, the food suppliers now need to match supplies to the nutrient requirements of the community. This means that food policy should be geared to the provision and consumption of foods of the quality and in the quantities that are necessary to promote and sustain nutritional health and to reduce the risk of developing the diseases discussed in this report.

The chronic diseases that may be prevented by providing an adequate diet fall into two broad categories: those due to insufficient food and those due to an excessive intake of certain foods or nutritional components (the toxic effects of food contaminants are not included in this analysis). Nutritional deficiencies can now no longer be considered simply as those (e. g., protein–energy malnutrition or iron deficiency anaemia) that are prevalent in developing countries. In developed countries the "affluent" diet is deficient in complex carbohydrates derived from cereals, tubers, and pulses; these together with vegetables and fruits provide important ingredients, including dietary fibre, that have now been linked to the prevention of such conditions as cancer, as well as constipation. Deficiency diseases are also still found in vulnerable groups, e. g., children, pregnant women, and the elderly, within developed countries, so that nutritional deficiencies then coexist with the diseases caused by an "affluent" diet. It is now clear that both nutritional problems also coexist in the developing world.

Combating deficiency diseases in the developing world requires a range of strategies that have evolved over several decades and are well documented in a number of reports (e. g., *1, 4, 55*). They include the prevention and management of communicable diseases, income distribution schemes, and production and distribution strategies aimed at improving food supplies, economic development, and the welfare of the population.

However, very different strategies are required in both developed and developing countries to prevent the diseases associated with an "affluent" diet; these are the strategies of particular concern in this report. It is important, however, to ensure that there are no conflicts (which may be more or less difficult to resolve) between the two sets of strategies. Such conflicts can arise, for example, if a reduction in salt intake is advocated when salt is used as a vehicle for iodine or fluoride for the prevention of iodine deficiency or dental caries.

6.2 Establishing policies in the 1940s

Nutrition and food policies were formulated in many developed countries more than 50 years ago when there was concern about the quantity and quality of the diet being consumed by the general public. With the discovery of vitamins, the importance of protein, and the role of minerals and other micronutrients, it was important to ensure that the population's diet was varied and well balanced. The consumption of only a limited range of foods is more likely to lead to a deficiency state since few foods are rich sources of all the nutrients. Analyses of different foods revealed that meat and dairy products were a major source of protein and provided substantial amounts of calcium, iron, zinc, and other micronutrients, including the B vitamins. Feeding trials also showed that children, particularly if small for their age, grew faster if fed extra milk, so great emphasis was placed on ensuring that there was a plentiful intake of animal products.

The remarkable increase in understanding in the 1930s of the role of vitamins, minerals, and protein in maintaining health was not confined to the developed world. In a number of developing countries it was recognized that beriberi, pellagra, scurvy, xerophthalmia, goitre, and many other conditions could be relieved by the provision of adequate intakes of micronutrients. The description of nutrient deficiencies in the developing world highlighted the importance of nutrition and amplified the concern of public policy-makers in both affluent and developing countries to provide a well balanced and adequate diet. The rigours of the Second World War demanded exceptional measures to ensure food supplies, and these, combined with pervasive health education campaigns, were remarkably successful in maintaining the health of sections of affluent communities living under highly stressful conditions. Only when food blockades or widespread war devastation occurred did malnutrition become evident, so the authorities became convinced that the problems of nutrition in affluent societies could be tackled and that the major problem was one of ensuring a good supply of nutrients and a plentiful intake of animal products.

Authorities in the developed world therefore sought to maximize the production of meat and milk. Economic policies that included large subsidies, support for marketing initiatives, controls on animal-feed prices, standards for meat-carcass quality, and minimum milk-fat content all developed in conjunction with major educational programmes through, for example, the schools, medical services, and the media. The public was also led to believe that the quality of milk and meat is related to its fat content, especially "good" sources of food being butter and cream.

As a result, a large part of the agricultural industry in many affluent countries is geared to providing cereals, pasture, or other feeds for animal production, and to producing meat and milk. Furthermore, most governments still see this sector of the industry as in need of promotion, even if animal feeds have to be imported. Thus, over decades, affluent countries have striven to produce more meat and milk, and this policy continues to dominate much of agricultural thinking in Eastern and Western Europe.

The developing world has also been influenced by this thinking. Protein–energy deficiency was described in Africa, and then in the Caribbean, during the 1940s and this condition was soon identified as widespread by nutritional research workers throughout the world. Recurrent famines, endemic vitamin deficiencies, and the nutritional emphasis on protein deficiency as a cause of kwashiorkor led to intense efforts by governments and international agencies to improve the diet of rural communities and to encourage animal production where possible.

It is, thus, not surprising that in most, if not all, developing countries government policies have been established to promote or modify the home production or sale of food, but it is very rare for any of these policies to have a nutritional basis designed to cope with the principal concerns of this report. The ability to feed a country's population is accepted as a primary responsibility of governments, but practically all government actions are now geared to economic or political priorities, such as maintaining the economic state of rural communities, providing cheap food for urban populations, or controlling the import/export trade to ensure an appropriate balance of payments. This approach recognizes the importance of improving the standard of living of the large rural populations, as well as that of the rapidly expanding urban communities. More complex policies have also been developed to improve food security, i. e., a population's ability to feed itself in years with bad harvests or bad weather conditions. These measures may include adjustments in taxation, improved facilities for storage, buffer stocks of food, or the construction of roads to ensure easier distribution of food stocks from one part of the country to another.

Thus the main priorities of government planners and administrators dealing with food policy are related to the economic and political issues of food availability and cash crops, with little attempt so far to deal with current nutritional issues. The economic planning is, in fact, based on an understanding of nutrient needs as defined in the 1940s and 1950s. It is against this background that governments in the developing world will need to consider how best to develop nutrition and food policies if they wish to avoid a progressive rise in the incidence of chronic diseases in their countries.

There has been a widespread tendency to oversimplify nutrition policies and to assume that many nutritional problems can be solved by an expansion of animal production. The need to reconsider agricultural and food priorities is not helped by the fact that economic, marketing, and farming practices were established in accordance with the old food policies. There are entrenched farming and industrial interests that will not welcome the reduced emphasis on milk and meat production, and a policy specifying the wisdom of consuming only modest amounts of meat and milk low in fat content. Many farming policies have also been developed to encourage the cultivation of sugar beet and sugar cane as a method of supporting farm incomes. Sugar as a commodity has the advantage of being readily transported and non-perishable. It is not surprising, therefore, that large industrial interests in affluent societies are now involved in maintaining or promoting sugar consumption.

The activities of many governments are dominated by economic issues, and agriculture has been developed over several decades not only to provide enough food for the population, but also to ensure that the farming community's viability and welfare are maintained at a reasonable level. In many developed countries, e. g., in North America and Europe, and in Japan, there are substantial financial subsidies for farmers. Agricultural policy is therefore a very important issue in any discussions on trade, and these economic issues understandably have high priority in government planning. The dilemma for those in the field of public health is that, although the nutritional thinking of 50 years ago led to a sense of urgency as regards the improvement of agriculture, the priorities set then have been incorporated into routine government policy-making without specific concern for nutritional objectives. The relatively new philosophy concerned with the prevention of chronic diseases is only now beginning to emerge as an issue in agricultural policy in developed countries, and has not been considered before by agricultural economists and planners in the developing world. Since the new nutritional objectives of preventing both the deficiency diseases and the chronic diseases of the developed world may have immense implications for the economics of farming, government industrial and social policies, and international trade, it will inevitably take time for coherent policies and programmes to emerge, and for entrenched attitudes to change. The following section deals with the experiences of individual countries and regions, before an attempt is made to draw conclusions from early attempts to develop or modify national nutrition and food policies.

6.3 Regional food policies in Europe

6.3.1 *Background*

An overview of food policies that were created originally in response to the nutritional concerns of the 1930s and 1940s can be considered on a regional basis. But it must be recognized that within any one region there may be remarkable variations in policy linked to the climatic, geographical, social, cultural, and political conditions of individual countries.

One example of the development of a food policy may serve, however, to illustrate the way in which coordinated government action, initiated by nutritional concerns 50 years ago, developed in such a comprehensive manner that adjustment to cope with our current understanding of nutritional needs is not easy. In the United Kingdom, substantial grants were made originally to develop the dairy industry; milk marketing boards were established to facilitate the production, distribution, and sale of milk, with guaranteed prices for milk and butter production. These boards improved the bargaining power of the farmers and their financial returns. Prices were linked to the level of fat in the milk, and high-quality milk was identified as that with a particularly high fat content. Daily delivery of milk and other dairy products to individual households was instituted on a national scale and became part of the social fabric of society, providing a guaranteed source of milk, eggs, cream, and butter to the elderly, infirm, and isolated. Government controls on carcass-grading ensured that fattened sheep and cattle received special subsidies.

Since the Second World War, there has been a remarkable growth in the food industry in Europe as well as in North America. The progressive increase in the numbers of women at work, and the desire for convenience foods, have stimulated further demands for food that can be processed and packaged for a long shelf-life, and for simple serving and cooking in the home. Thus, in some countries over three-quarters of all food purchased is now packaged and/or processed in one way or another. Supermarket chains that retail food have also grown rapidly to provide a convenient way of purchasing a wide variety of foods of good quality at a reasonable price.

Over the last 10 years, there has been a tendency for consumers to demand leaner meat and a major disparity has developed between the amount of animal fat produced by the European farmers and consumers' purchasing preferences. Unwanted surplus animal fat has therefore often been produced with the help of the government subsidies that were originally introduced to increase meat and dairy production. This surplus fat has then understandably been used by food manufacturers to produce a wide variety of cheap food products that are rich in fat. Competition is fierce among the supermarket chains, and food manufacturers, with traditionally some of the lowest profit margins of any industry, have no alternative but to attempt to produce ever cheaper food. Over several decades, there have therefore been substantial changes in the types of food product made available in the shops. In northern Europe, this has often resulted in a change in the pattern of fat intake, with a reduction in "visible" fat consumption and an increase in the consumption of "invisible" fat in food products. Also, it is often not recognized that many governments have legal and financial constraints on producing lean meat and lower-fat milk; this problem has only been tackled by a few countries. The constraints often take time to identify and evaluate, because they have become part of the normal processes of national economic management.

A similar shift in sugar consumption is apparent in many countries, with consumers seeking to reduce their sugar consumption for health reasons only to find that this cheaply produced commodity is being used widely to provide a cheap and attractive component of a wide range of food products.

In many countries, the public's perception of a high-quality diet as abundant in animal products and rich in fat has been sustained by decades of public education, as well as by a cultural acceptance that these foods were at one time luxury items in the diet of the poor. This persisting view can now present problems. Governmental controls on farming, or attempts to persuade the population of the virtues of a low-fat intake from meat and milk, can be unpopular if advice is seen to be given for economic rather than health reasons. Thus, in some Eastern European countries, the popular demand for more foods of animal origin is a big political issue. Most governments do not yet recognize that the current medical-scientific views on diet and health can also be economically advantageous, since there is no longer the need to produce such large quantities of meat and milk or to feed cattle in ways that produce fatty carcasses. Farming policies that do not require intensive animal production systems would also reduce the world demand for cereals; a very large proportion of international trade in cereals is for animal feed. Cereal importation for animal production, which today is a drain on foreign currency in many Eastern European countries, would no longer be a priority if grass feeding with slower cattle growth were to become acceptable. This, in turn, would mean that the use of land could be reappraised, since cereal production for direct consumption by the population is much more efficient and cheaper than dedicating large areas to growing feed especially for cattle production and dairying. Nevertheless, in many Eastern European countries, the population considers the ready availability of large quantities of meat and milk at a reasonable price a desirable feature of an affluent life-style. This emphasizes the complex nature of any programme to help a population achieve a healthier way of life.

6.3.2 Health promotion and the roles of producers and manufacturers

In several Western European countries and in North America, there have been sustained public education campaigns, either by the government or by major medical charities, that aim to change the public's eating pattern. These campaigns usually compete with the much greater advertising campaigns for individual foods by food companies. These companies could play an important part in developing new foods with a more appropriate nutrient content, but advertising for foods rich in fats, sugar, and salt continues so that company profitability can be maintained. This legitimate concern is also linked to the claim that modest intakes of the products are still compatible with a healthy diet and that all an individual company is doing is maintaining its market share. Since most or all food companies can reasonably use the same argument, it is clear that it is the responsibility of government, the medical profession, and consumer organizations to consider the overall impact of unfettered promotion of food products. Unfortunately, the idea that medical opinion is divided and that policies are uncertain is often used to inhibit change, despite the remarkable consistency of views put forward by expert groups over several decades (see Annex 4).

Farmers are not necessarily resistant to change; traditionally they express social concern since they value their image as responsible contributors to society. Some food manufacturers may not yet have developed a similar concern, but the majority of food manufacturers in Europe are small and based locally, and may be receptive to new ideas on nutritional requirements. Food producers and processors sometimes differ in their attitude to new public health demands that may not have industrial logic. In theory, farmers have the greater problems of adjustment, but the widespread governmental support given to farmers throughout Europe since the Second World War (in research, development, and advice) may have contributed to their flexibility. Farmers have revolutionized their agricultural practices over the last 40 years in response to the demands for greater food production and seem willing to change again. In comparison, there has been little research and development by government research institutions for the food industry. With the relatively low involvement in research and development of the food industry itself it is not surprising that the industry is less used to change and will need much more help. Currently, its priorities are to introduce new technologies for food processing, with only limited attention being given to improving the nutritional quality of food products.

6.3.3 *Controls on marketing*

In some countries, there are agreed policies to limit the advertising of confectionery and alcohol during children's radio and television programmes, but an evaluation of the long-term impact of advertising on the public's perceptions of food quality and health has rarely been attempted. Given the widely recognized dangers of tobacco use, there are increasing moves to limit both the advertising of cigarettes and sports sponsorship by tobacco companies, despite the intense lobbying to prevent these developments. To adopt the same policies for foods would be more difficult because governments and the public have yet to accept, for example, that saturated fatty acids are as hazardous to health as smoking. Given the wide variety of foods rich in these fats, agreement would be required on the level of saturated fatty acids that would warrant restrictions on advertising. So far only generic controls, e. g., on confectionery advertising to children, have been introduced and the extension of this policy would meet opposition. Nevertheless, labelling of foods to allow the nutrient content to be readily recognized is being widely considered. This would help consumers and teachers to educate children in appropriate eating habits (see below).

6.4 Experiences of promotion of healthy diets in some developed countries

Experiences of the promotion of healthy diets in Europe have recently been assessed by the World Health Organization Regional Office for Europe (*74*), and some of the examples given in that publication, as well as others concerning North America and Australasia, will be given here.

6.4.1 *Finland*

Finland had the highest rate of heart disease in the world in the period after the Second World War and was chosen to participate in the Seven Countries Study conducted by Keys and his colleagues. This study led to the emphasis on serum cholesterol and dietary saturated fatty acids as causal factors in the development of coronary heart disease.

130

In Finland, the province of North Karelia had the highest death rate from heart disease and the community consequently demanded that preventive action be taken long before the medical profession considered the evidence sufficient to warrant action. Local political initiatives led to a major community-based campaign involving schools, the media, public education, and numerous lay organizations. Despite the dominance of farming in the region, especially dairy farming, substantial changes in diet occurred, with the introduction of low-fat milks and alternative, vegetable, sources of fats rich in polyunsaturated fatty acids. The methods used for promoting health have been described (75), but the debate continues about whether this selective action in North Karelia was really responsible for the observed decline in heart disease (76). Throughout Finland there was an increased awareness of nutrition and health promotion, accompanied by a countrywide decline in death rates.

In 1985, the Finnish parliament charged the Inter-Ministerial Advisory Board on National Food and Nutrition Supply to develop national dietary recommendations and a comprehensive food policy by 1990. This work is now under way and involves the food producers and food manufacturers.

6.4.2 The Netherlands

In response to consumer interest, the parliament, in 1981, requested the Netherlands Nutrition Council to issue guidelines for a healthy diet. In 1984, a comprehensive nutrition report was adopted as a policy by the Netherlands parliament, with emphasis on food safety as well as health, and in 1986, dietary guidelines were established, including nutrient goals. The policy document and the guidelines recommended the surveillance of dietary patterns and the institution of a food consumption survey; this was carried out in 1987 and the first report was published in 1988. A central data bank was developed to allow the collation of up-to-date information on the nutrient composition of new foods being introduced, especially those aimed at helping people with food allergies. The policy paper, as well as the guidelines, underline the need to reduce the population's fat intake, and especially the consumption of saturated fatty acids. Since these developments are recent, it would be too early to expect any change yet in the rates of heart disease.

6.4.3 *Norway*

Norway is unusual in having published dietary recommendations for the prevention of cardiovascular diseases as early as 1963. In 1975, the Norwegian parliament also adopted a nutrition and food supply policy to link agricultural policy with health-promoting activities. Norway has a much more limited range of farming options than the United States and Australasia, because the northern, cooler climates are more conducive to farming grass than to cereal or fruit production. The dependence of farmers on ruminant production from grass, i.e., the raising of dairy and beef cattle and sheep, is therefore understandable and there were some conflicts between the farmers and the health promoters, which the parliament's policy sought to resolve. Norwegian agriculture is heavily dependent on subsidies and the government has emphasized national food self-sufficiency, by attempting to promote cereal and vegetable growing. Price adjustments have been used to encourage changes in farm practice, but the financial support to farmers for traditional food products continues to be very high.

The Ministry of Social Welfare has always been responsible to parliament for monitoring nutrition policy. Since 1982, greater emphasis has been given to health promotion, with nutrition education of the public. With government-initiated action, the fat content of the Norwegian diet fell from over 40% in 1975 to 36% in 1988. Death rates from ischaemic heart disease have also fallen, by 14% in males and 23% in females from 1970 to 1985, but this is modest compared with the decreases observed in Australasia, Canada, and the United States of America (*77*).

6.4.4 *The United Kingdom of Great Britain and Northern Ireland*

The United Kingdom responded to new concepts of diet and health by issuing qualitative guidelines in 1974 advocating a reduction in fat and sugar intakes. The advice was couched in cautious terms compatible with the scientific doubts of the experts who analysed the relationship between diet and health. No action was taken by the government or the health authorities, other than the issue of a pamphlet, with a small circulation, on healthy eating.

In 1976, quantitative dietary guidelines were produced by the Royal College of Physicians along the lines of many of the reports of national and international expert groups. Explicit dietary advice was given, but again the report had little public impact. Community physicians involved in the preparation of the report, however, established a voluntary organization, the Coronary Prevention Group, to inform the government and public about the need for change in life-style. Several concerned physicians then began a public campaign by means of radio, television, and lecturing, despite the intense opposition of many physicians and nutritionists whose perceptions were still based on the dietary requirements to avoid deficiency diseases. A National Advisory Committee on Nutrition Education was then formed by the government's Health Education Council and the food industry's British Nutrition Foundation and produced quantitative guidelines in 1983 (78). The government also produced quantitative guidelines in 1984, in effect accepting the international scientific consensus on the role of diet in cardiovascular disease. More recently, an independent national audit office has called for a coherent programme for preventing chronic diseases (79). Almost all health districts have now adopted their own local food and health policies; there is intense consumer interest and the media give thorough coverage to any novel development in healthy nutrition or food safety. Dietary patterns are changing rapidly, particularly among the more affluent sections of society. The original claims by food manufacturers that they were already catering for consumer needs were soon proved wrong when national promotion of low-fat milk led to its immediate uptake by 20% of the market, with a marked increase in sales of other low-fat products. Confusion continues, however, about the nutritional content of processed foods in the absence of any uniform comprehensive food-labelling system.

The farming and economic policies are of course linked to those of the European Economic Community, and are not necessarily in line with current concepts of diet and health. About 75% of the population of all ages eat more than the limit advised by government of 35% of energy from fat, and the distribution of serum cholesterol levels is so high that at least two-thirds of adults require immediate dietary advice on the basis of the standards set by the European Atherosclerosis Society.

Despite these impediments to change, some parts of the United Kingdom are now involved in specific programmes of health promotion, the most coherent being "Heart-Beat Wales", which involves public education, lay groups, schools, factories, retailers, and many other groups. The Health Education Authority has also launched a government-backed "Look after your heart" campaign.

The United Kingdom has seen only a very small improvement in health, with a 10% fall in coronary heart disease death rates in men over the last 20 years, and a 2% fall in women. The United Kingdom, together with Finland and Ireland continues to be at the top of the world table for deaths from heart disease. It also has one of the highest rates of breast and large bowel cancer, and more than 50% of its middle-aged population are overweight.

6.4.5 *The United States of America*

One of the first countries to engage in a public health campaign to lower intakes of fat and saturated fatty acids was the United States of America. In 1963, the American Heart Association initiated a campaign that soon gained substantial publicity. This foundation is a voluntary organization specifically set up both to help those with heart disease and to promote preventive measures. The population was very health conscious; health care was the responsibility of the individual, people choosing their own doctors and medical specialists according to their needs and ability to pay. This may explain the readiness with which the population sought and accepted new concepts for health promotion and altered their life-styles accordingly. Thus the reduction in smoking, the increase in exercise, and the emphasis on dietary changes to limit increases in serum cholesterol were apparent among the educated groups in society in the USA before they were observed elsewhere. The interest in diet and preventive measures intensified, with doctors often having to respond to the demands of their patients for information and advice at a time when the medical profession was untrained in both nutrition and the newer concepts of prevention. The demand for information led to the formation of self-help groups. A number of local schemes were initiated involving community physicians, consumer organizations, and other lay groups. The government responded by providing information but the limited number of government controls and the continued use of agricultural subsidies to promote sugar, milk, and beef production meant that government decision-making was not involved in the campaigns for prevention.

The USA has seen a reduction of over 40% in the death rate from coronary heart disease and there has been much discussion about the causes of this change. One analysis, based on the effects of risk changes and on the recognized benefits of medical therapy, coronary bypass operations etc., suggested that about 40% of the observed decline in death rates could be attributed to medical intervention, 30% to the reduction in serum cholesterol, and 24% to the reduction in smoking. Thus, over half the effect was ascribed to changes in lifestyle. The average fat content of the diet in the USA continues to be high and obesity is very prevalent, but objective indices of adipose tissue stores of fatty acids, e. g., linoleic acid, indicate quite clearly a progressive change in the level of fatty acids that correlates closely with the decline in death rates from heart disease. The consumption of lean meat, low-fat milks, and vegetable oils low in saturated fatty acids has become widespread and may explain the decrease in the national average serum cholesterol levels and the decline in heart disease. Thus in a period of eight years, from 1977 to 1985, the intake of low-fat milk increased by 60%, and this in part accounted for 33% of women having fat intakes below 35% energy by 1985, compared with about 25% of British women. The population in the USA continues to be highly health and diet conscious, with one popular health magazine having sales of 10 million copies per month. The general population is also very aware of the significance of an elevated serum cholesterol level. The public in the USA continues to "manage" its own health in certain respects, with 58% of women taking supplements of vitamins or minerals in 1985. These women also tend to be those on a more satisfactory diet and can therefore be considered particularly health conscious.

6.4.6 *Australasia*

Australia and New Zealand have also benefited from a substantial decline in heart disease. Both countries are major exporters of agricultural produce including meat and dairy products, but their climates are also conducive to cereal, vegetable, and fruit production. Health consciousness is high, a variety of government health campaigns have been under way for many years, and there are few legal or economic reasons that might hinder farmers wishing to respond to consumer demands. The free market economies ensure a rapid response to consumer demand, but this demand has depended on the effectiveness of public health education. This has necessarily been presented alongside other campaigns that attempt to promote foods and beverages that are high in fat, sugar, salt, or alcohol. It is noteworthy that, despite this confusion, there have been substantial decreases in ischaemic heart disease in Australia and New Zealand between 1970 and 1985, in both men and women, by between 31% and 51% (77).

6.5 Food strategies in developing countries

Food and nutrition policies in the developing world have focused primarily on food production, the control of communicable diseases, and education. In disaster-prone areas especially, the main focus has been necessarily on maintaining national food availability. It is only in countries where sufficient food is available for all that other strategies have been designed for equitable distribution. Table 15 summarizes the emphasis given in developing food policies in 21 developing countries. It is noteworthy that none of the policies had a specific nutritional objective, and most policies were dominated by issues of producer welfare and self-sufficiency.

Implicit and explicit food and nutrition policies were developed, however, in several countries. Implicit policies were formulated, for example, in Costa Rica, Cuba, and Panama, and explicit food policy statements and food planning initiatives were made in Brazil, the Caribbean countries, Colombia, Honduras, the Philippines, and Thailand, among others. Food production policies have also been made explicit in a number of African and Asian countries.

In recent years, increased emphasis has been given to developing regional strategies for food security, i.e., the ability to withstand temporary food shortages (81). Examples of such arrangements include those of the Cartagena Agreement Board (JUNAC, Junta del Acuerdo de Cartagena) in the Andean region, the Association of South East Asian Nations (ASEAN) in southern Asia, and the Caribbean Community (CARICOM). Although there have been many failures, a number of countries have benefited greatly from these policies.

It is now well accepted that food policies have to move away from short-term crisis management to plans for sustainable improvements in food availability. These plans of action may include interventions in taxation, credit, trade and exchange rates, and agricultural prices and controls, and measures to distribute benefits and incentives. Timmer et al. (82) have identified various interventions aimed at ensuring food security and improving diet and nutrition status (Table 16). Their list is not exhaustive, but illustrates interventions that may be selected as part of a food strategy. Nutritional

Table 15. Government food policy objectives for 21 developing countries [a]

Country or area	Consumer welfare	Producer welfare	Government revenue	Foreign exchange	Self-sufficiency	Stable prices	Food security	Specific nutrition objective [b]
Africa								
Botswana		×			×		×	
Kenya		×		×	×		×	
Mali		×			×	×		
Morocco					×			
Nigeria		×			×			
Senegal		×			×			
Sudan		×		×	×			
United Republic of Tanzania					×			
Asia								
Bangladesh	×	×		×	×	×	×	
India	×	×			×	×	×	
Indonesia	×	×			×	×	×	
Philippines		×			×	×	×	
Sri Lanka	×	×			×	×		
Thailand	×	×	×	×		×		
Latin America								
Brazil	×			×	×			
Dominican Republic	×			×	×			
Guatemala	×	×	×	×	×	×	×	
Haiti		×					×	
Jamaica		×						
Paraguay		×		×				
Peru	×	×					×	

× indicates that this type of objective is specified.
[a] Adapted by FAO from reference 80; reproduced by kind permission of the Food and Agriculture Organization of the United Nations.
[b] No specific nutrition objectives were identified.

interventions are normally implemented separately, and usually seek to identify vulnerable subgroups within society.

It is now recognized that dietary deficiencies cannot be solved simply by increasing food production or by educational programmes. The socioeconomic level of the population is also of major importance, so it is necessary to assess the production, marketing, and consumption of food, as well as the social and economic factors conditioning them. To provide for "food security" requires an analysis of the extent of rural development, the adequacy, quality, and safety of food production, rural access to food and trade, external food aid, and international trade. National food and nutrition policies therefore need to coordinate policies taken in each individual area.

Table 16. Categories of intervention included in food strategies [a]

	Food security	Diet and nutrition status
Targeted	Food stamps, with a means test [b]	Maternal and child health clinics, with a means test
	Fair-price shops, with a means test and/or geographical or commodity targeting	Nutrition education; weaning foods
	Targeted rationing programmes	Vitamin and mineral supplements for deficient populations
	Supplementary feeding programmes for vulnerable groups	Malnutrition wards in hospitals for severe cases
	Price subsidies for specific food commodities	
	Food-for-work programmes	
Not targeted		
Direct	General food rationing schemes	Nutrition education on radio and television and through other general media
	Fair-price shops for primary foodstuffs, with unrestricted access	General fortification schemes (for example, iodized salt)
Indirect	Adjusted exchange rate for imported food	Encouraging breast-feeding; discouraging infant formula
	General food price policy or subsidy	Public health interventions (water, sanitation, inoculations)
	Food production input subsidies (fertilizer, water, credit, seed, machinery)	

[a] Adapted from reference *82*, by kind permission of the World Bank.
[b] A means test is a measure of financial assets and income, with lower prices being paid by those with lower income.

A strategy may include short- and long-term measures. Scarce resources and political considerations may necessitate short-term measures such as increasing price support for the producer, raising import subsidies, or the fortification of foods. Investments in infrastructure, for example, in warehouses, buffer stocks, and roads, may require large amounts of foreign exchange but have beneficial effects in the long term. Both producer and consumer interests should be considered and arrangements should be made so that a balance is struck within a clearly defined time-frame. Finding the right policy mix is always a compromise.

The failure of some food strategies is illustrated by the wheat policy followed in one Latin American country. The effects of high prices paid to the producer, designed to increase local production as a substitute for imports, were offset by concomitant consumer subsidies. These consumer subsidies, once established, proved difficult to remove because vested interests supported their continuation. Exchange-rate changes also led to higher prices for wheat imports so the consumption of imported wheat by the poor was made more difficult. Yet improving the access of the poor to wheat was the original objective of the increase in producer prices. This underlines the complex social and economic implications of using price policies to safeguard food consumption and nutrition.

The implementation of effective strategies is also constrained by the lack of financial resources. This budgetary restriction has been a major factor in forcing many countries to re-evaluate their policies and interventions in the food system. For example, food subsidies have been a primary instrument of government policy in many countries, but, because of the economic downturn in the 1980s, subsidies are now being reduced or eliminated in the process of structural adjustment. Possible reforms include the liberalization of grain markets, encouraging privatization, and increasing incentives by raising prices paid to producers. Price reforms on their own can have only modest effects, because productive resources and inputs, infrastructural changes, technological development arising from agricultural research and extension, post-harvest services, macro-economic factors, and the weather are other limiting factors.

Smallholders are very responsive to price reforms, but other changes, including institutional reforms, are needed to give small farmers a minimum purchasing power. Low-income groups can also increase their own food production or can be helped (but less effectively) if food surpluses are made available at reduced prices. Improving food availability for the poor, therefore, can involve increases in their incomes, the use of subsidies, or food aid. Targeting subsidies for the poor may reduce the financial burden on the national government, but targeting may be expensive and fraught with administrative problems. Sometimes these pressures may be minimized by devising self-targeting mechanisms—by placing subsidies on less prestigious foods which are bought only by the poor. Most food and nutrition policies do not tackle either the main underlying cause of undernutrition, i.e., a lack of purchasing power, or the rising levels of nutrition-related disease.

The health sector has an important role in food security that is often poorly understood. Family planning contributes significantly in the medium term to the total amount of food, or purchasing power, available both to the family and nationally. Food hygiene, personal hygiene, and the prevention of infectious diseases also limit the waste of nutrients. The promotion of breast-feeding and food hygiene also increases the availability of food within the household by limiting illness.

6.6 Examples of interventions by selected countries

In India and Pakistan there are restrictions on international trade and on movement across state borders, and these measures tend to increase the prices in poor areas. In the Republic of Korea, however, producer price support, including credit and input subsidies, is a policy designed to increase self-sufficiency and the equality of urban and rural incomes. Consumer subsidies appear to be the most widely adopted policy instrument, but most countries also maintain government control over cereal imports, as well as the retail prices of wheat and rice, because of the growing importance of wheat and rice in urban diets. A targeted subsidy, in the form of food stamps, is currently provided in Sri Lanka and the USA, but unless the stamps can be exchanged for a fixed quantity of food their value to the recipient can be eroded by inflation.

African governments have tended to establish government monopolies by means of parastatal organizations that are responsible for the procurement and marketing of cereals, and the distribution of other foods or subsidy systems. Government agencies in Asia also have these functions, but they have emphasized large public food-distribution programmes designed to target low-income consumers. In South America support mechanisms vary; Brazil and Paraguay have subsidized credit to influence production, whereas other countries in the region have relied primarily on official prices paid to the producer.

Many governments are now becoming aware of the need to ensure the nutritional quality of the diet as well as its microbiological and toxicological safety. New concepts in nutrition, e.g., in relation to the fat content and composition of vegetable oils, such as coconut, palm, and soya-bean oils, are also now important for agricultural exports from developing countries. This is partly because of the scale of economic dependency that many countries have on the revenue earned from agricultural food exports, and also because in developing countries themselves, there is a new concern for the health of their urban populations as diet-related chronic diseases become more of a health problem. For example, in China it is now recognized that economic reforms will influence food production and consumption, and with the object of guiding food production and consumption in a way that will benefit the health of the public, the Chinese Government has announced that food and nutrition policy will be one of its major concerns in the coming years. The policy and planning issues related to food and nutrition that are under consideration in China include the impact of the national plan for agricultural production (including price policies on both food production and consumption); the implications of economic strategies for food imports and exports, the food laws and regulations for the food-processing and food-service industries, and the influence of food industries and marketing on food habits are also considered. The consequences for health of the emerging dietary patterns of the urban and rural population groups, and the need to have adequately trained personnel to deal with these issues at central as well as at provincial level are also recognized.

6.7 Conclusions based on preliminary attempts to promote healthy nutrition in a modern context

Is it possible to discern a set of key principles for action from these varied national experiences? Clearly the economic policies of governments vary widely and the health care systems are very different. The traditions for tackling public health problems related to nutrition range from an almost exclusive concentration on public education to a perception that the availability, price, and nutrient composition of foods are a major responsibility of the national government and will have a profound effect on food and nutrient consumption. This last view was held by many governments during the Second World War and remains an accepted principle in many countries. Nevertheless, several conclusions clearly emerge from the brief summaries of national experiences presented in this section:

1. Government economic policies affecting food production, processing, distribution, and sales, if specifically organized to promote food production, are often based on outmoded ideas about what constitutes a healthy diet. As such they may be an impediment to dietary change and health promotion.
2. Once a public health problem has been identified by a government, or by medical research workers, major changes in dietary behaviour are rarely promoted by the medical profession. Indeed, the medical profession often lags behind public demand for health-promoting measures. Nevertheless, its knowledge,

understanding, and promotion of new concepts in healthy nutrition could provide an important stimulation to community change.

3. The greater the consumers' sense of responsibility for their own health, the greater the speed of behavioural change, e.g., in diet, smoking, and exercise. Populations with access to a free health care system that is effective and widely available for treating disease may be more inclined to rely on medical advice and less likely to initiate behavioural changes themselves.

4. Despite the apparent confusion in dietary messages in many developed countries, and the advertising of foods high in fat, sugar, and salt, a reasonably well educated public seems able to distinguish these contradictory messages from information on prevention given by health promoters and unbiased sections of the media. Nevertheless, the slower rate of change in life-style seen among the less affluent and less well educated may reflect the impact of these contradictory promotional efforts. The initiation and maintenance of successful health promotion campaigns often seem to depend on voluntary organizations or on small groups of activists.

5. Preventive measures have not had a high priority with any government. Few health departments yet have the effective working relationships with other departments involved in food production, e.g., agriculture, trade, and finance, that will be needed when an integrated nutrition and food policy is introduced.

6. Following health promotion initiatives at the national level, there seems to be a delay of at least five years before appreciable changes are observed in national statistics on health and disease, even though special studies show that definite dietary changes can lead to rapid effects. Most European initiatives have only begun within the last five years and initiatives in many regions of the world have not yet started.

7. In developing countries, the need to develop a nutrition and food policy appropriate to prevention of the chronic diseases observed in affluent societies is a high priority, because the current economic planning (including agricultural policies, subsidies, etc.) may adversely affect the health of the community over the next 5–10 years.

These conclusions, and knowledge of the effect of the health promotion campaigns and nutrition policies of 50 years ago, led the

Study Group to propose a new set of actions appropriate to both the developed and the developing world.

6.8 New proposals

6.8.1 *Factors needed for successful nutrition and food policies*

Many non-nutritional factors can lead to the success or failure of nutrition and food policies. Consequently, in addition to being physiologically sound, they must be politically viable, economically feasible, and culturally acceptable. To achieve this, food and nutrition policies must have the credibility provided by scientific and epidemiological evidence, have political and technical support, and be regarded as necessary and convenient by the consumer. All this indicates that the development and implementation of food and nutrition policies require multisectoral government actions. These actions need to be coordinated to be effective; they should involve the whole food chain, from the production or importation of food through to its consumption.

Sustained determination over many years is needed to implement a nutrition policy. It must also be recognized that the prevention of diet-related chronic diseases requires a broad approach that goes beyond the food production-consumption chain. It involves government action on smoking, and policies to encourage leisure-time physical activity, to combat poverty, to provide a hygienic environment, and to combat communicable diseases.

Some of these problems are more difficult to tackle than others. Difficulties often arise with deficiency diseases in developing countries, where there may be acute social and economic problems that lead to political instability. This can be illustrated by the slowness or inability of the health authorities to reduce infant malnutrition in many countries. Paradoxically, some of the countries that do not have adequate public health policies in relation to infant malnutrition do have financial and technical resources that would allow them to embark on a prevention programme relating to chronic diseases, and some governments have expressed an interest in dealing with these problems. Some of the issues relating to healthy diet may therefore be simpler to handle than the elimination of protein–energy deficiency, for example.

6.8.2 *The multisectoral and multidisciplinary approach*

The development and implementation of food and nutrition policies in a country require the participation of government sectors involved in health, agriculture, economics, education, social welfare, planning, and development, all of them with support from the highest levels of decision-making. Technical or operational assistance should be provided by the nutrition community, universities, and nongovernmental organizations interested in health and social development, and, in many cases, also by the food industry, farmers' organizations, the catering industry, and others.

Cultural and social acceptance of the policy by the population is crucial. Community leaders, educators, communicators, marketing specialists, anthropologists, and other social scientists may be needed to ensure that the implementation of the policy is made in a way that benefits the consumer. In most countries consumers are aware of the relationship between good nutrition and health, and this awareness must be stimulated and developed whenever possible. The importance of involving consumer organizations and voluntary organizations based within the community cannot be over-emphasized.

6.8.3 *Formulating specific nutrition and food policies*

The details of a suitable nutrition and food policy to prevent chronic diseases and promote healthy nutrition will vary according to each country's political, cultural, social, and economic circumstances, the health of its population, the possibilities of producing or importing foods and food ingredients, the diseases that are to be prevented, and the characteristics of the target population groups.

It is suggested, on the basis of experience in several countries, that a board or council for nutrition and food policy should be established by the government to allow a fully integrated approach to the prevention of chronic diseases. This will need to draw on many government departments and disciplines to be fully effective.

It is inappropriate to set out in this report the means by which a nutrition board might operate. In centrally managed economies, the responsibilities of the board should be established in a manner that will allow the government processes relating to food production, distribution and sale, trade policies, economic policy, and educational systems to be integrated with health concerns.

In countries where the political and economic structure is different, the development of a board should be considered within the national context. Effective nutrition policies require coordinated action by many ministries, so the challenge is to develop effective means of interacting on health issues, when non-health concerns have priorities that may be different from those of the ministry of health. It is suggested that if the climate of public opinion on health can be changed first, through education and community involvement, then a change can be made in political priorities and in turn in governmental action. It is understandable that financial matters such as import/export policies are considered without thought to any health implications. Once a society has been convinced, however, by community and media involvement that there are important health or environmental factors to be coped with by some change in economic priorities, then it is surprising how rapidly public opinion can change and lead to subsequent government action. Ministries of health should not, therefore, rely solely on intragovernmental discussions to achieve policy changes, because in most societies government decision-making on its own has only modest effects on community life-style, unless drastic measures are taken. In some countries, the ministry of health is also seen to be a relatively ineffective department when it comes to influencing general government policy-making. Thus, the dual approach of promoting an awareness of the health issues through involving the public and the simultaneous holding of discussions with other government departments should be recognized as an effective mechanism for achieving changes in government policy-making.

Fig. 20 displays some of the interactions that are needed in both the formulation and the implementation of a nutrition and food policy. In the figure, the ministry of health is shown separately to emphasize the point that the ministry of health need not wait for the formulation of an interdepartmental mechanism for interchange and planning before it takes action.

It is suggested that a fundamental role of the nutrition and food board should be to involve nongovernmental organizations and consumer representatives. In many developing as well as developed countries there are cancer societies, cardiac societies, and special interest groups, such as women's groups, who can play a valuable role in developing policy. It is therefore best to include them at the earliest possible stage in the process of policy-making, as well as in policy implementation.

146

Fig. 20. Formulating a nutrition and food policy

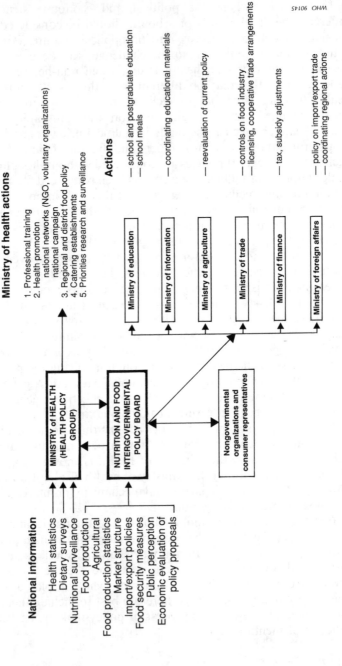

Ministry of health actions

1. Professional training
2. Health promotion
   national networks (NGO, voluntary organizations)
   national campaign
3. Regional and district food policy
4. Catering establishments
5. Priorities research and surveillance

Actions

Ministry of education
— school and postgraduate education
— school meals

Ministry of information
— coordinating educational materials

Ministry of agriculture
— reevaluation of current policy

Ministry of trade
— controls on food industry
— licensing, cooperative trade arrangements

Ministry of finance
— tax, subsidy adjustments

Ministry of foreign affairs
— policy on import/export trade
— coordinating regional actions

MINISTRY of HEALTH (HEALTH POLICY GROUP)

NUTRITION AND FOOD INTERGOVERNMENTAL POLICY BOARD

Nongovernmental organizations and consumer representatives

National information

Health statistics
Dietary surveys
Nutritional surveillance
Food production
Agricultural
Food production statistics
Market structure
Import/export policies
Food security measures
Public perception
Economic evaluation of policy proposals

6.8.4 *Initiatives and proposed responsibilities of the ministry of health*

Three fundamental types of information should be collected by the ministry of health, which will need a group of officials who are well versed in nutritional issues so that they can undertake responsibility for data collection and policy analysis:

—the current state of, and trends in, the nutritional status of the population;
—health statistics relating to nutritionally linked diseases; and
—data on the current state and trends in food supply plus, if available, dietary survey data.

Nutritional status
The ministry of health may already have a mechanism for monitoring the nutritional status of the population. If so, then it should consider how best to extend the surveillance so that it takes account of the new needs in relation to nutrition policy-making. Ideally, nutritional surveillance should include:

1. *Monitoring a random sample of the adult population for obesity and risk factors for coronary heart disease,* i.e., body weight, height, serum cholesterol levels, and hypertension rates. It would be useful to obtain data on tobacco use and alcohol intake at the same time. This need not be an expensive process, and samples of, say, 100–200 adults of each sex in both urban and rural areas will provide a developing country with preliminary information to alert the ministry of health to any major problems. Data can readily be handled for this size of sample, and repeating the survey at perhaps yearly intervals will allow any trends to be distinguished. Measuring adult weight and height has often been seen as a low priority, but can provide invaluable information on the problems of chronic energy deficiency as well as obesity. It also serves as a primary tool for estimation of the population's energy requirements. How to do this has been set out recently by James & Schofield (*69*).

2. *Monitoring children's weight and height.* This serves the dual purpose of alerting ministries of health to changing rates of growth and growth failure, as well as indicating whether obesity is appearing among the general population. Monitoring the prevalence of communicable diseases is also useful in developing

countries, since these may also result in growth failure and inadequate intake of food in a proportion of the population.

3. *Monitoring anaemia.* This can readily be done by analysing blood samples used for measuring serum cholesterol. A decision to assess the prevalence of anaemia in children should also be made in the light of local knowledge. This knowledge may also demand special investigations of specific nutrient deficiencies.

4. *Monitoring salt intake.* This is best done by collecting and analysing 24-hour urine specimens from a random sample of subjects.

Health statistics

Health statistics should be collected from a variety of sources. Special small surveys may be needed to assess the validity of mortality and morbidity statistics. In developed countries, a variety of techniques have been advocated for these purposes. Collating data on health provides invaluable information not only for formulating strategies but also for explaining the needs for new policies to the public and to government.

Data on food supply and consumption

Food balance-sheet data provided by FAO can give valuable information about levels and trends in the food supply. If national, food balance sheets exist, they usually provide more accurate information. Although not specifically providing data on the nutritional state of children and adults, dietary surveys in one form or another may also play a crucial part in establishing both the likely risk of nutrient deficiency and how the dietary pattern is changing. Food consumption data are fundamental to the formulation of an integrated nutrition and food policy. Dietary data need to be sufficiently detailed to allow the intakes of children, adults, and the elderly to be assessed separately. There are many reports on the various ways of obtaining data on food supply and consumption (*83, 84*).

Nutrition policy objectives and nutrient targets

To guide the implementation of nutrition and food policies, governments will have to formulate clear policy objectives. These may be given at a general level, or specifically, as in the case of nutrient targets that can be achieved within a defined period of time. Examples of such nutrient intake targets have been set out in a book published by the WHO Regional Office for Europe (74). These incorporate ultimate targets, as well as intermediate nutrient intake targets, such as those chosen by several northern European countries. A further example is that of China, where it was recently decided to use an intermediate target of 10 g of salt per person per day as a national average, since the current intake is estimated to be approximately 17 g per day.

Intermediate nutrient intake targets should be developed by ministries of health after consultations with other government departments. Depending on the structure of the administration, this decision-making may be incorporated into the government's general policy-making, but it is important that experts in medicine, epidemiology, nutrition, and agricultural economics are all involved in making an analysis of the costs and benefits of setting an intermediate target. It should also be recognized that the implications of working towards an intermediate target may be quite different from those of achieving the ultimate nutrient goals. For example, if the levels of total fat or saturated fatty acid intake were very high, then the food industry in that country could be asked to produce food products with a lower fat content and this would lead to a considerable reduction in the importation of fats and oils. Achievement of the ultimate goal might require a programme of fundamental agricultural change, which might take several decades to carry out.

In addition to an evaluation of current food consumption, it is also very useful to identify, where possible, trends in food consumption, because if some are beneficial from the nutrient goal point of view, then these trends can perhaps be readily amplified by appropriate government action, e.g., by health education or by removing economic barriers that may be limiting the availability of the food or increasing its price.

Trends in food availability and population trends may also make it possible to make some projections. These could be important not only for agricultural development but also from the health point of view. For example, in China, it is expected that despite a substantial increase in population by the year 2000—to 1.3 thousand million —cereal intakes will rise from 400 million tonnes to 500 million tonnes, and that cereal availability will remain at about 400 kg per caput per year. Clearly, if cereals come to be used for animal production or for fermentation to alcohol, this would have marked effects on cereal availability for direct consumption by the population. Alternative sources of food, e.g., fats and sugars, would then need to be considered in relation to the nutrient goals, and utilization of these would herald an adverse trend in diets. Therefore, by understanding the trends in food consumption, it is sometimes possible to foresee likely problems that may arise in the next 5–10 years.

6.8.5 *Policy development: the formation of food goals*

Policy should, ideally, be developed by the nutrition and food board but, in its absence, the ministry of health can initiate the process by developing food goals.

Food goals (i.e., goals relating to the consumption of specific foods, such as vegetables, fruit, meat, and dairy products) are clearly needed if the public is to gain an understanding of the practical significance of policies whose object is to ensure that a population's average nutrient intake moves towards the "ideal" *nutrient goal* shown in Table 13 (page 108). Food supply and consumption data will provide invaluable information on the per caput food intake or availability. On this basis, it will be evident which foods provide the nutrients of principal concern to the community. Some sensitivity and collaboration will be required, however, in drawing up food goals, since agricultural interests will clearly be involved if the food pattern proposed implies substantial change. Interaction between government departments will also be needed to ensure that the government does not inadvertently promote adverse trends in community dietary patterns.

Food goals need to be considered with great care and in relation to the agricultural policy and economic opportunities of the country. There may be options that agricultural experts could devise to meet the needs of both the consumer and the farming community. There is little evidence so far of agricultural experts being involved in the preparation of a nutrition and food policy, except in so far as they assume that the goal is to produce more food with certain classic qualities, e.g., an adequate protein content and a minimum of toxicants and antinutritional factors.

The factors affecting food production, availability, and price are many, and it would clearly be beneficial to consider each of these. Care must be taken, however, to ensure that the analysis is not prolonged. Without a fairly rigid time schedule for decision-making, a government may well find that dietary trends and previous government policies are already establishing consumer patterns of eating that are disadvantageous. A timetable for considering government changes is therefore essential when the mechanism for ensuring intersectoral exchange is established.

The variety of options for setting food goals within one country is great and country-by-country differences preclude a global analysis of the issues in this report. Nevertheless, the nutrition policy objectives are clear and the challenge now is how to deal with the implications for food needs. Several examples have been presented in this section of the different mechanisms governments have adopted for coping with the need for a nutrition policy. Annex 6 considers some of the issues involved in the development of a meaningful food-labelling scheme that can readily be understood by consumers.

6.8.6 Implementation of a nutrition and health policy by the ministry of health

There is no longer any need to compartmentalize action on the prevention of chronic diseases. Given the concordance in views on the dietary pattern needed to prevent cancer, to minimize the effects of obesity, to prevent diabetes, to cope with hypertension in the community, and to prevent coronary heart disease, it is now possible to pool resources at the government level so that effective initiatives in prevention can be sustained. In an earlier WHO report on the community prevention and control of cardiovascular diseases (40), it was suggested that the ministry of health should play a crucial role by:

—developing national action plans;
—encouraging community organization for health education;
—supporting youth involvement in education;
—promoting use of the mass media in the community-based health education programmes;
—defining the role of (a) the physician, (b) other health personnel, and (c) medical and other voluntary organizations; and
—developing demonstration projects.

Details may be obtained from the earlier WHO report (40), but one central theme emerges from the analyses of earlier efforts to develop an effective community-based prevention programme: it is essential to involve the community at every stage in the process of

151

implementing a nutrition policy. The mechanisms by which this can be done need to be carefully considered. Thus, it is of little value to initiate a centrally directed public health campaign if the community, for a variety of reasons, is culturally used to regarding government action as of little value to the individual's welfare. Intrinsic cynicism of the motives of some government programmes should not be underestimated, so it is important to enlist the support of independent voluntary bodies, including the nongovernmental organizations. This can be done in three ways:

1. Voluntary organizations could be provided with the background information needed to enable them to develop a community-based programme for the prevention of chronic diseases. This should include health statistics, results of dietary studies, and an evaluation of the nutritional status of the community, so that they can understand the background to the policy. Although there is a natural tendency for governments to work out an implementation strategy on their own and then to invite the voluntary organizations to comment on it, experience from countries governed by a wide variety of political systems suggests that an early involvement of voluntary organizations has immense advantages. The organizations are automatically enlisted in the implementation process and learn to understand the problems the government is trying to tackle. In general, voluntary organizations that are seen by the community as least likely to be influenced by general government policy-making are the ones whose help it is most important to enlist. Thus, a voluntary organization should be chosen on the basis of its community involvement rather than because of its earlier experience of participation in government advisory committees or other government processes. The voluntary organizations can also be asked to undertake preliminary analyses of the community's attitude to the prevention programme and how it might best be implemented. This approach would provide invaluable information to the ministry of health, and open up a major channel for transferring information and opinion throughout the community.

2. Voluntary organizations could be invited to participate at an early stage in advising the government on the best way of coping with the many problems that will be encountered when implementing an effective nutrition and food policy. In general,

governments that favour the use of experts only, while neglecting the need for intelligent representation of consumer or patient interests, are least effective in their health promotion schemes. Experts in medical research, nutrition, and epidemiology may be cautious when involved in government advisory roles and may not have a clear view of what is needed for community action. This limits their value once the stage of implementing policy is reached.

3. The ministry of health might consider how best to ensure that voluntary organizations operate effectively in an independent capacity. Many voluntary organizations provide sophisticated and independent representation of important sectors of public opinion, but they may be poorly funded and unable to operate effectively. Some ministries of health have therefore provided modest sums of money to voluntary organizations in order to ensure their viability and capacity to undertake work of value to the community. A balance needs to be struck between encouraging the participation of voluntary organizations and allowing them to remain unbiased representatives of their sectoral interests and independent of government.

Experience in both developed and developing countries has repeatedly emphasized the value of unofficial systems for warning the government of the ineffectiveness of policy implementation at the community level, and of the actual or perceived problems being encountered in converting nutrition education into practice. Voluntary organizations can also adequately reflect the cultural pressures that it is important to take account of in the implementation process.

6.9 Use of the mass media

The national mass media have a major role to play at all stages of health promotion. Their complete involvement therefore needs to be ensured by bringing them in at an early stage in the development of the new nutrition policy. Representatives of the mass media can make a major contribution to this policy-making process, and care should be taken to avoid the concept emerging that government officials and medical or nutritional experts are responsible for the policy-making and that the mass media should only later be involved in the task of transmitting the conclusions and decisions to the public. If leaders of the mass media are involved at an early stage, they come to learn the importance of a particular set of nutrients and of food goals and are better able to influence their colleagues so that a balanced message can be conveyed to the public.

The ministry of health in countries where the government controls the radio and televison should take steps to ensure that other sections of the mass media, e.g., newspapers, magazines, and trade journals, are also involved, so that the public perceives the information to be of relevance to them, as well as beneficial to the government's policy-making process. Mass-media experts trained in behavioural sciences and practised in the skills of health communication need to be included in the health promotion efforts. Ministries may find it useful to support a group of mass-media experts who can assess the best way of amplifying community action. These experts have many skills that are often unrecognized by medical personnel and need to be used to the full. The development and production of educational material suitable for presentation by the mass media needs to be carefully considered, and there are now well established principles for producing such material (85).

The mass media, when involved in community programmes, often find that effective change can best be developed by concentrating on a specific set of needs within a community, rather than by simply providing a broad campaign on the need for a healthy life-style. When the mass media are involved in the promotion of health education, they frequently demand the involvement of medical experts who must be willing to acquire and use the communications skills suitable for mass-media presentation. The experts also have responsibility for ensuring that mass-media personnel are fully aware of the medical basis for the prevention programme.

6.10 Professional training and involvement

The ministry of health should approach professional organizations to ensure their involvement in initiating change within the medical profession. Medical education will need to change in many countries to include instruction, demonstration projects, and the development of skills in disease prevention. Education should include some knowledge of the behavioural sciences, in particular information relevant to both individual and community change. The professional organizations should be asked to encourage community physicians and general practitioners, in particular, to take a leadership role in developing a community-based programme for the prevention of chronic diseases. A professional organization can also be asked to see how best to initiate the changes in attitude needed if ideas on medical care are dominated by a demand in the community for effective therapeutic advice and management. If physicians can play a leading role, this will help to promote the active participation of the whole health care team in a multifaceted community-based prevention programme. The wide range of personnel involved should be recognized, e.g., nurses, pharmacists, dentists, health educators, public health personnel in factories, offices and the retail trade, as well as health personnel involved in schools and in the community care of the sick, infirm, and elderly.

Many countries in both the developed and developing world have found that the professionals, e.g., doctors, nurses, teachers, and community workers, are uncertain of their role in preventing chronic diseases because their training has not prepared them for this. Postgraduate as well as undergraduate training is an essential component of the overall strategy, because the demands of prevention cannot wait for a new generation to be trained. The ministry of health can help promote a sense of urgency by involving the professional organizations in developing postgraduate education suitable for implementation and effective action by health professionals within the next 5–10 years.

Experience has suggested that preventive measures at the national level, and the involvement of nongovernmental and other voluntary organizations as well as the mass media, should not be delayed until the professionals are confident that they can respond to a public demand for help. The driving force for community behavioural change is often community-based, and it is often at the level of primary health care that the medical professions find an active role in prevention despite being under pressure to maintain their therapeutic services. A community demand for help may be an important stimulus, and lead to local self-help schemes, developed for example in conjunction with community health centres and other areas of community action such as schools.

6.11 Demonstration projects

Demonstration projects within the medical delivery system are also valuable. The network of health services throughout the country provides an ideal opportunity for demonstrating the importance that the ministry of health attaches to the prevention of chronic disease. Thus, in designating the criteria to be used in feeding staff in hospitals, it is important to create an appropriate environment, in which smoking is discouraged and where exercise can be taken. In these and many other ways, the ministry of health can have, itself, a substantial impact on the community, because of the interactions that these individuals have at so many levels with the medical delivery system. Workers at all levels within the health services should also be of primary concern to the ministry of health. Before any community-based demonstration projects are developed, it is possible for government action to have a direct effect by promoting good practices and setting standards for future community developments.

Demonstration projects were discussed in an earlier report on the control of cardiovascular disease (40). In summary, they provide an opportunity to demonstrate the control of disease through preventive measures at the local level and to develop cost-effective methods of health education. The importance of interaction between different groups within the community becomes evident and can provide an important resource at the national level for assessing the overall effectiveness of preventive measures. These projects also serve as a centre for training and for assessing the needs for improving the health promotion process.

6.12 Evaluation and monitoring

Early attempts to develop disease-prevention programmes show that it is important to develop a monitoring scheme to ensure that such programmes are conducted effectively. With so many organizations involved, it is very easy to believe that progress is being made in making the public aware of the issues. However, the most effective measure for achieving changes in behaviour, and then promoting the alterations in diet necessary for preventing disease, have to be developed on the basis of objective criteria of success. Without adequate monitoring of the extent to which the community understands the problem, of how the community is implementing change, and of how much change has taken place, the ministry will be unable to evaluate its programme. A programme or campaign will then, if ineffective, prove to be counterproductive as organizations become disenchanted with the response to their efforts. It is important, therefore, that the nutrition and health policy group should monitor regularly the amount of information that is being transmitted to the community and how it is being used.

Comprehensive national monitoring schemes have been established in some developed countries, but this may not be possible in many less affluent societies. An effective way of obtaining information is to conduct regular small surveys of the work of health personnel, of community involvement in prevention programmes, of community knowledge of nutrition, and of behavioural change. In this way the ministry of health can adjust to changing community needs without establishing an elaborate structure of surveillance.

7. CONCLUSIONS

Dietary factors are now known to influence the development of a wide range of chronic diseases, e.g., coronary heart disease, various cancers, hypertension, cerebrovascular disease, and diabetes. These conditions are the commonest cause of premature death in developed countries and they impose major burdens on society. On current projections, cardiovascular diseases and cancer will emerge, or be established, as substantial health problems in virtually every country in the world by the year 2000.

The "affluent" type of diet that often accompanies economic development is energy-dense. People consuming these diets characteristically have a high intake of fat (especially saturated fats) and free sugars and a relatively low intake of complex carbohydrates (from starchy, fibre-containing foods). Such diets are well established in developed countries, and are now becoming more common in most developing countries, where they are typically adopted first by the urban, upper- and middle-class population. This change in diet can now be linked to the increasing incidence of chronic diseases and of premature death. Evidence suggests that many of these premature deaths and disabilities should be preventable by changes in diet and in other aspects of life-style. Governments and communities, in both developing and developed countries, should act now to reduce the future burden of these diseases. Their prevention or reduction is both a social responsibility and an economic necessity.

Because of the diversity and complexity of diets in different countries, of local food supplies, and of the social, economic, and political contexts in which changes of national diets are to be sought, this report does not prescribe detailed policies and strategies. It proposes, as a general approach, a population-oriented primary prevention strategy, based on national nutritional goals, and employing broadly based intersectoral policies that include a food and nutrition policy. It also stresses the need for greater emphasis on health in the formulation of agricultural policies, and of economic, import/export, employment, and education policies.

A rational public health policy should seek to influence the national diet in the direction of the population nutrient goals elaborated in section 5. These nutrient goals are population averages (see Table 13, page 108); they specify, for each nutrient, the range within which the average per caput intake should lie. Changing the national diet to achieve these goals, and maintaining patterns of nutrient intake within these recommended ranges, will yield maximum health benefits.

The nutrient goals indicate that the health needs of the population are best met by a high-carbohydrate, low-fat diet, rich in starchy foods (e.g., cereals, tubers, and pulses) and including a substantial intake of vegetables and fruit. Only small quantities of essential fats are required. While the protein content of most national diets is already adequate, continuing attention must be paid to the problems of maldistribution of protein-containing foods within some countries, and to the protein needs of young children in developing countries.

In many developing countries, the authorities must continue to deal with a range of nutritional deficiencies within at least some segments of their population. However, governments and other bodies in developing countries should act now to prevent increases in incidence of the chronic diseases that will accompany an inappropriate diet. They have the opportunity to intervene before the typical dietary patterns traditionally associated with affluence become widespread and established within their populations. In formulating interventions, governments in developing countries should identify the indigenous plant foods that are of high nutritional value, and should encourage their production and consumption. Further, the local food industry should be encouraged to develop processing techniques that do not add fat, sugar, or salt to food products.

8. RECOMMENDATIONS

8.1 Recommendations to WHO

The Study Group recommended that WHO should consider:

1. Developing a coherent nutrition and health policy with targets for promoting the concept of healthy nutrition. This concept, which supplements the long-standing concern with nutritional deficiencies and food shortages, takes account of the increased risks of chronic diseases in later adulthood caused by the "affluent" dietary pattern (i.e., high in fats and free sugars, and low in starchy foods) that tends to accompany economic development.
2. Establishing a mechanism to ensure that the impact of diet upon a range of health problems is recognized in all relevant WHO programmes.
3. Discussing with other United Nations and international agencies the major implications for agriculture and trade of the nutritional needs of both developing and developed countries, as described in this report. Commodity analyses and the projections of FAO should be considered in relation to the nutritional quality of the diet.
4. Communicating to the major trading organizations the consequences of trading developments that might lead to adverse effects on health. The export of subsidized saturated fat is an example of one potential problem.
5. Strengthening its programme to provide expert guidance to national governments seeking to establish a nutrition and food policy, for example by means of seminars for national governments and nongovernmental organizations.
6. Developing a basis for monitoring the progress of the initiatives described in this report on diet and health, and setting targets for this work. In this regard the development of surveillance programmes at country level should be promoted.
7. Discussing with nongovernmental organizations how best to ensure that communities throughout the world participate in activities to promote health by eating an appropriate diet. The variety of diets consistent with the nutritional goals should be recognized, and the nutritional goals translated into food needs at national level.

8. Monitoring research developments and promoting international collaboration in the study of the relationships between diet and health so that further refinements to the Organization's nutrition policy can be made.
9. Involving the Codex Alimentarius Commission[1] in establishing standards that will help to implement the proposals in this report.

8.2 Recommendations to national governments

10. Governments are recommended to establish a national board for nutrition and food policy involving, in addition to the ministry of health, the many government ministries whose policies affect the production, distribution, and consumption of food.
11. Governments should ensure that experts are available to the ministry of health to monitor the nutritional and health status of the population, as assessed by a national surveillance system.
12. Ministries of health should initiate or strengthen professional training programmes, at both undergraduate and postgraduate levels, to ensure that the role of diet in the prevention of chronic diseases is understood by the medical profession and other health care workers.
13. Each ministry of health should, as part of its health promotion programme, establish regular contact with nongovernmental organizations, consumer representatives, and the media to develop jointly a community-based programme. This activity should be in addition to any government-sponsored health promotion campaign.
14. Governments should ensure that adequate nutritional competence exists within the ministry of agriculture to allow full participation in a national board for nutrition and food policy.
15. Governments should consider their investment and subsidy policies in both agriculture and the food industry to ensure that they are consistent with the nutritional concepts contained in this report. Policies should be geared to promoting the growing of plant foods, including vegetables and fruits, and to limiting the promotion of fat-containing products.

---

[1] The Codex Alimentarius Commission is an intergovernmental body with a membership, in 1989, of 137 countries; it is charged with the implementation of the FAO/WHO Food Standards Programme.

16. As part of a national policy, each government should set its own goals and strategy for reducing the incidence of chronic diseases.
17. Governments are recommended to establish appropriate food standards, to ensure the nutritional quality of foods that are substantial contributors to the national diet.
18. Each government should consider all new legislation bearing on agriculture and food, to ensure that it is compatible with the prevention of chronic diseases.
19. Governments are recommended to establish, where possible, compulsory labelling of food products based on the Codex Standards and Guidelines for the Labelling of Foods and Food Additives.[1] Labelling should be clear and consistent and, to be understandable as well as scientifically correct, information should be simply presented and expressed both graphically and numerically. One method is proposed in Annex 6.
20. Discussions should be encouraged between the government, the food industry, and the consumers to ensure the development of food products that are low in fat, free sugars, and salt.
21. Each government should examine its animal production policies and incentives to ensure that they do not promote the production of excessive quantities of saturated fats.
22. Ministries of education should ensure that, as part of nutrition and health education for teachers and children, due attention is given to the prevention of diet-related chronic diseases.

ACKNOWLEDGEMENTS

The Study Group wishes to acknowledge the valuable contributions made to its work by: Dr K.V. Bailey, Regional Officer for Nutrition, WHO Regional Office for Africa, Brazzaville, Congo; Dr H.W. Heiss, University of Freiburg, Freiburg, Federal Republic of Germany; Dr E. Helsing, Regional Officer for Nutrition, WHO Regional Office for Europe, Copenhagen, Denmark; Dr F.K. Käferstein, Chief, Food Safety, WHO, Geneva, Switzerland; Dr E. Nicholls, Regional Adviser, Noncommunicable Diseases, WHO Regional Office for the Americas, Washington, DC, USA; and Dr R. Saracci, Unit of Analytical Epidemiology, International Agency for Research on Cancer, Lyon, France.

---

[1] CODEX ALIMENTARIUS COMMISSION. *Codex Alimentarius, Volume VI. Codex Standards and Guidelines for the Labelling of Foods and Food Additives*, 2nd ed. Rome, Food and Agriculture Organization of the United Nations/World Health Organization, 1987.

REFERENCES

1. *The fifth world food survey*. Rome, Food and Agriculture Organization of the United Nations, 1987.
2. HETZEL, B.S. The control of diseases related to nutrition. In: Holland, W.W. et al., *Oxford textbook of public health*. Oxford, Oxford University Press, 1983, vol. 4, pp. 22–46.
3. DEMAEYER, E.M. Xerophthalmia and blindness of nutritional origin in the Third World. *Children in the tropics*, **165**: 2–33 (1986).
4. UNITED NATIONS ADMINISTRATIVE COMMITTEE ON COORDINATION—SUBCOMMITTEE ON NUTRITION. *First report on the world nutrition situation*. Rome, Food and Agriculture Organization of the United Nations, 1987.
5. DEMAEYER, E.M. & ADIELS-TEGMAN, M. The prevalence of anaemia in the world. *World health statistics quarterly*, **38**: 301–316 (1985).
6. FAO Food and Nutrition Series, No. 23, 1988 (*Requirements of vitamin A, iron, folate and vitamin B_{12}*: report of a Joint FAO/WHO Expert Consultation).
7. MURRAY, J.J., ed. *Appropriate use of fluorides for human health*. Geneva, World Health Organization, 1986.
8. LITVAK, J. ET AL. The growing noncommunicable disease burden, a challenge for the countries of the Americas. *Bulletin of the Pan American Health Organization*, **21**(2): 156–171 (1987).
9. GURNEY, M. & GORSTEIN, J. The global prevalence of obesity—an initial overview of available data. *World health statistics quarterly*, **41**: 251–254 (1988).
10. NISSINEN, A. ET AL. Hypertension in developing countries. *World health statistics quarterly*, **41**: 141–154 (1988).
11. INTERSALT COOPERATIVE RESEARCH GROUP. Intersalt: an international study of electrolyte excretion and blood pressure. Results for 24 hour urinary sodium and potassium excretion. *British medical journal*, **297**: 319–328 (1988).
12. *World population prospects 1988*. New York, United Nations, 1989 (Population Studies No. 106).
13. *Evaluation of the strategy for health for all by the year 2000. Seventh report on the world health situation*. Volume 1. *Global review*. Geneva, World Health Organization, 1987.
14. WORLD BANK. *World tables*, 3rd ed. Vol. I, *Economic data*. Washington, DC, Johns Hopkins University Press, 1983.
15. *World agricultural statistics*. Rome, Food and Agriculture Organization of the United Nations, 1986.
16. BURKITT, D. & TROWELL, H. *Refined carbohydrate foods and disease. Some implications of dietary fibre*. London, Academic Press, 1975.
17. GU, X.Y. & CHEN, M.L. Vital statistics, health services in Shanghai County. *American journal of public health*, **72**: 19–23 (1982).
18. POBEE, J.O.M. The status of cardiovascular disease in the setting of disease of environmental sanitation and hygiene and malnutrition: the West African (Ghana) experience. In: Lauer, R.M. & Shekelle, R.B., ed. *Childhood prevention of atherosclerosis and hypertension*. New York, Raven Press, 1980.
19. SINNETT, P. ET AL. Social change and the emergence of degenerative cardiovascular disease in Papua New Guinea. In: Alpers, M. & Attenborough, R., ed. *Human biology of Papua New Guinea: the small cosmos*. Oxford, Oxford University Press (in press).

20. *World population trends, population and development interrelations and population policies, 1983 monitoring report.* Volume 1. *Population trends.* New York, United Nations, 1985 (Population Studies No. 93).

21. GOLDMAN, L. & COOK, E.F. The decline in ischaemic heart disease mortality rates: an analysis of the comparative effect of medical intervention, and changes in lifestyle. *Annals of internal medicine,* **10**: 825–830 (1984).

22. HAYDEN, B. Subsistence and ecological adaptations of modern hunter/gatherers. In: Harding, R.S.O. & Teleki, G., ed. *Omnivorous primates: gathering and hunting in human evolution.* New York, Columbia University Press, 1981, pp. 344–421.

23. MCKEOWN, T. *The role of medicine: dream, mirage or nemesis.* London, Nuffield Provincial Hospitals Trust, 1976.

24. COHEN, L. Diet and cancer. *Scientific American,* **257**(5): 42–48 (1987).

25. BOYDEN, S. *Western civilization in biological perspective. Patterns in biohistory.* Oxford, Oxford University Press, 1988.

26. GOPALAN, C. Dietary guidelines for affluent Indians. *Bulletin of the Nutrition Foundation of India,* **9**(3): 1–4 (1988).

27. *Dietary guidelines and nutrition policies in Japan.* Tokyo, Japan Dietetic Association, 1984.

28. KEYS, A., ed. Coronary heart disease in seven countries. *Circulation,* **41**(suppl. I): I-1–I-211 (1970).

29. KEYS, A. ET AL. The seven countries study: 2289 deaths in 15 years. *Preventive medicine,* **13**: 141–154 (1984).

30. KEYS, A. *Seven countries: a multivariate analysis of death and coronary heart disease.* Cambridge, MA, Harvard University Press, 1980.

31. WHO Technical Report Series, No. 678, 1982 (*Prevention of coronary heart disease*: report of a WHO Expert Committee).

32. SHAPER, A.G. ET AL. Alcohol and ischaemic heart disease in middle aged British men. *British medical journal,* **294**: 733–737 (1987).

33. DAYTON, S. ET AL. A controlled clinical trial of a diet high in unsaturated fat in preventing complications of atherosclerosis. *Circulation,* **40**(suppl. II): II-1–II-63 (1969).

34. MIETTINEN, M. ET AL. Effect of cholesterol-lowering diet on mortality from coronary heart disease and other causes. A twelve-year clinical trial in men and women. *Lancet,* **ii**: 835–838 (1972).

35. STAMLER, J. & SHEKELLE, R. Dietary cholesterol and human coronary heart disease: the epidemiological evidence. *Archives of pathology and laboratory medicine,* **112**: 1032–1040 (1988).

36. FAO Food and Nutrition Paper, No. 20, 1977 (*Dietary fats and oils in human nutrition*: report of a FAO/WHO Expert Consultation).

37. WHO Technical Report Series, No. 628, 1978 (*Arterial hypertension*: report of a WHO Expert Committee).

38. WHO Technical Report Series, No. 686, 1983 (*Primary prevention of essential hypertension*: report of a WHO Scientific Group).

39. WHO Technical Report Series, No. 715, 1985 (*Blood pressure studies in children*: report of a WHO Study Group).

40. WHO Technical Report Series, No. 732, 1986 (*Community prevention and control of cardiovascular diseases*: report of a WHO Expert Committee).

41. MACMAHON, S. ET AL. Blood pressure, stroke, and coronary heart disease. Part 1, prolonged differences in blood pressure: prospective observational studies corrected for the regression dilution bias. *Lancet,* **335**: 765–774 (1990).

42. COLLINS, R. ET AL. Blood pressure, stroke, and coronary heart disease. Part 2, short-term reductions in blood pressure: overview of randomised drug trials in their epidemiological context. *Lancet*, **335**: 827–838 (1990).

43. NATIONAL RESEARCH COUNCIL COMMITTEE ON DIET, NUTRITION AND CANCER, ASSEMBLY OF LIFE SCIENCES. *Diet, nutrition, and cancer*. Washington, DC, National Academy Press, 1982.

44. US DEPARTMENT OF HEALTH AND HUMAN SERVICES, PUBLIC HEALTH SERVICE. *The Surgeon General's report on nutrition and health*. Washington, DC, US Government Printing Office, 1988 (Publication No. 88-50210).

45. NATIONAL RESEARCH COUNCIL. *Diet and health: implications for reducing chronic disease risk*. Washington, DC, National Academy Press, 1989.

46. DOLL, R. & PETO, R. *The causes of cancer*. Oxford, Oxford University Press, 1981.

47. *Alcohol drinking*. Lyon, International Agency for Research on Cancer, 1988 (IARC Monograph on the Evaluation of Carcinogenic Risks to Humans, Vol. 44).

48. CARROLL, K.K. Experimental studies on dietary fat and cancer in relation to epidemiological data. In: Clement, I.P., et al., ed. *Dietary fat and cancer*. New York, Alan R. Liss, 1986, pp. 231–248.

49. ROYAL COLLEGE OF PHYSICIANS. Obesity. A report of the Royal College of Physicians. *Journal of the Royal College of Physicians of London*, **17**(1): 5–65 (1983).

50. BENDER, A.E. & BROOKES, L.J., ed. *Body weight control: the physiology, clinical treatment and prevention of obesity*. Edinburgh, Churchill Livingstone, 1987.

51. LEW, E.A. & GARFINKEL, L. Variation in mortality by weight among 750 000 men and women. *Journal of chronic diseases*, **32**(8): 563–576 (1979).

52. GARROW, J.S. Indices of adiposity. *Nutrition abstracts and reviews, series A*, **53**(8): 697–708 (1983).

53. JAMES, W.P.T., ET AL. Definition of chronic energy deficiency in adults. *European journal of clinical nutrition*, **42**: 969–981 (1988).

54. NATIONAL CENTER FOR HEALTH STATISTICS. *Anthropometric reference data and prevalence of overweight. United States 1976–1980*. Hyattsville, MD, Department of Health and Human Services, 1987 (Publication No. (PHS) 87–1688; National Health Survey Series 11, No. 238).

55. WHO Technical Report Series, No. 724, 1985 (*Energy and protein requirements*: report of a Joint FAO/WHO/UNU Expert Consultation).

56. FRANÇOIS, P.J. *Prevalence of overweight within household and household diet (a Brazilian case-study)*. Rome, Food and Agriculture Organization of the United Nations/Brazilian Institute of Geography and Statistics, 1989 (unpublished FAO document).

57. WHO Technical Report Series, No. 727, 1985 (*Diabetes mellitus*: report of a WHO Study Group).

58. SNOWDON, D.A. & PHILLIPS, R.L. Does a vegetarian diet reduce the occurrence of diabetes? *American journal of public health*, **75**: 507–512 (1985).

59. RUGG-GUNN, A.J. & EDGAR, W.M. Sugar and dental caries: a review of the evidence. *Community dental health*, **1**: 85–92 (1984).

60. RIGGS, B.L. & MELTON, L.J. Involutional osteoporosis. *New England journal of medicine*, **314**: 1676–1686 (1986).

61. ROYAL COLLEGE OF PHYSICIANS. *Fractured neck of femur—prevention and management*. London, Royal College of Physicians of London, 1989.

62. LIEBER, C.S. *Medical disorders of alcoholism; pathogenesis and treatment.* Philadelphia, W.B. Saunders, 1982.
63. BARRISON, I.G. ET AL. Adverse effects of alcohol in pregnancy. *British journal of addiction,* **80**: 11–22 (1985).
64. WHO Technical Report Series, No. 550, 1974 (*Fish and shellfish hygiene:* report of a WHO Expert Committee convened in cooperation with FAO).
65. HALSTEAD, B.W. & SCHANTZ, E.J. *Paralytic shellfish poisoning.* Geneva, World Health Organization, 1984 (Offset Publication, No. 79).
66. *Aquatic (marine and freshwater) biotoxins.* Geneva, World Health Organization, 1984 (Environmental Health Criteria 37).
67. WHO Technical Report Series, No. 399, 1968 (*Microbiological aspects of food hygiene:* report of a WHO Expert Committee with the participation of FAO).
68. *Nairobi + 10 : mycotoxins 1987. (Report of the Second Joint FAO/WHO/UNEP International Conference on Mycotoxins held in Bangkok, Thailand from 28 September to 2 October 1987).* Bangkok, Food and Agriculture Organization of the United Nations, 1988.
69. JAMES, W.P.T. & SCHOFIELD, E.C. *Human energy requirements: a manual for planners and nutritionists.* Oxford, Oxford Medical Publications, 1990 (published on behalf of the Food and Agriculture Organization of the United Nations).
70. FAO Food and Nutrition Series, No. 20, 1980 (*Dietary fats and oils in human nutrition:* report of an Expert Consultation).
71. BASSEY, J. ET AL. Reasons for advising exercise. *Practitioner,* **231**: 1605–1610 (1987).
72. ROSE, G. Sick individuals and sick populations. *International journal of epidemiology,* **14**: 32–38 (1985).
73. KANNEL, W.B. & GORDON, T., ed. *Framingham Study, 16-year follow-up.* Section 26. *Some characteristics related to the incidence of cardiovascular disease and death.* Washington, DC, US Government Printing Office, 1970.
74. JAMES, W.P.T. ET AL. *Healthy nutrition: preventing nutrition-related diseases in Europe.* Copenhagen, WHO Regional Office for Europe, 1988 (WHO Regional Publications, European Series, No. 24).
75. PUSKA, P. ET AL. The community-based strategy to prevent coronary heart disease: conclusions from the ten years of the North Karelia Project. *Annual reviews of public health,* **6**: 147–193 (1985).
76. PYÖRÄLÄ, K. ET AL. Trends in coronary heart disease mortality and morbidity and related factors in Finland. *Cardiology,* **72**: 35–51 (1985).
77. UEMURA, K. & PIŠA, Z. Trends in cardiovascular disease mortality in industrialized countries since 1950. *World health statistics quarterly,* **41**: 155–178 (1988).
78. NATIONAL ADVISORY COMMITTEE FOR NUTRITION EDUCATION. *A discussion paper on proposals for nutritional guidelines for health education in Britain.* London, Health Education Council, 1983.
79. NATIONAL AUDIT OFFICE. *Report by the Comptroller and Auditor General. National Health Service: coronary heart disease.* London, Her Majesty's Stationery Office, 1989.
80. USDA ECONOMIC RESEARCH UNIT. *Food policies in developing countries.* Washington, DC, 1983.
81. *Food security in food deficit countries.* Washington, DC, World Bank, 1980 (Staff Working Paper No. 393).

82. TIMMER, C.P. ET AL. *Food policy analysis.* Baltimore, Johns Hopkins University Press, 1983 (published for the World Bank).

83. BINGHAM, S.A. The dietary assessment of individuals; methods, accuracy, new techniques and recommendations. *Nutrition abstracts and reviews, series A,* **57**: 705–742 (1987).

84. BLACK, A.E. Pitfalls in dietary assessments. In: Howard, A.N. & McLean Baird, I., ed. *Recent advances in clinical nutrition.* London, J. Libbey, 1981, pp. 11–18.

85. FARQUHAR, J.W. ET AL. Education and communication studies. In: Holland, W.W. et al., ed. *Oxford textbook of public health.* London, Oxford Medical Publications, 1985.

Annex 1

RECOMMENDED DIETARY ALLOWANCES

Tables A1.1 to A1.4 summarize the recommended dietary intakes with respect to energy, protein, vitamins, and minerals.

Table A1.1. Daily average (per kg) energy requirements and safe level of protein intake for infants and children aged 3 months to 10 years (sexes combined up to 5 years)[a]

Age	Median weight (kg)	Energy requirement				Safe level of protein intake (g/kg)[b]
		(kcal$_{th}$/kg)		(kJ/kg)		
Months						
3–6	7.0	100		418		1.85
6–9	8.5	95		397		1.65
9–12	9.5	100		418		1.50
Years						
1–2	11.0	105		439		1.20
2–3	13.5	100		418		1.15
3–5	16.5	95		397		1.10
		Boys	Girls	Boys	Girls	
5–7	20.5	90	85	377	356	1.00
7–10	27.0	78	67	326	280	1.00

[a] Adapted from reference 1, Table 49, page 137.
[b] Minimum level considered safe.

Table A1.2. Daily average energy requirement and safe level of protein intake for adolescents aged 10–18 years[a]

Age (years)	Median weight (kg)	Energy requirement		Safe level of protein intake (g/kg)[b]
		(kcal$_{th}$)	(kJ)	
Boys				
10–12	34.5	2200	9 200	1.00
12–14	44.0	2400	10 000	1.00
14–16	55.5	2650	11 100	0.95
16–18	64.0	2850	11 900	0.90
Girls				
10–12	36.0	1950	8 200	1.00
12–14	46.5	2100	8 800	0.95
14–16	52.0	2150	9 000	0.90
16–18	54.0	2150	9 000	0.80

[a] Adapted from reference 1, Table 48, page 136.
[b] Minimum level considered safe.

167

Table A1.3. Daily average energy requirements and safe level of protein intake for adults[a, b]

| Weight (kg) | Energy requirement | | | | | | Safe level of protein intake (g/day)[c] |
	18–30 years (kcal$_{th}$)	(kJ)	30–60 years (kcal$_{th}$)	(kJ)	Over 60 years (kcal$_{th}$)	(kJ)	
Men							
50	2 300	9 700	2 350	9 700	1 850	7 700	37.5
55	2 400	10 100	2 450	10 100	1 950	8 300	41.0
60	2 550	10 600	2 500	10 400	2 100	8 600	45.0
65	2 700	11 300	2 600	10 900	2 200	9 100	49.0
70	2 800	11 700	2 700	11 200	2 300	9 600	52.5
75	2 900	12 300	2 800	11 800	2 400	10 000	56.0
80	3 050	12 900	2 900	12 000	2 500	10 400	60.0
Women							
40	1 700	7 200	1 900	7 900	1 650	6 800	30.0
45	1 850	7 700	1 950	8 300	1 700	7 100	34.0
50	1 950	8 200	2 050	8 500	1 800	7 500	37.5
55	2 100	8 600	2 100	8 800	1 900	7 900	41.0
60	2 200	9 200	2 200	9 000	1 950	8 200	45.0
65	2 300	9 800	2 250	9 400	2 050	8 500	49.0
70	2 450	10 300	2 300	9 600	2 150	8 900	52.5
75	2 550	10 800	2 400	10 000	2 200	9 300	56.0

[a] For a basal metabolic rate factor of 1.6.
[b] Adapted from reference 1, Tables 42, 43 and 44 (men) and Tables 45, 46, and 47 (women).
[c] Minimum level considered safe.

168

Table A1.4. Recommended dietary allowances of vitamins and minerals

Age	Vitamin A[a,b] safe level (µg retinol/day) M	F	Folate[a] (µg/day) M	F	Vitamin B12[a] (µg/day) M	F	Vitamin C[c] (mg/day) M	F	Vitamin D[c] (µg/day) M	F	Iron[a,d] absorbed (µg/kg per day) M	F	Zinc[e] (mg/day) M	F
Infants (months)														
0–3	350	350	16		0.1	0.1	20	20	10	10		120	3.1	3.1
4–6	350	350	24		0.1	0.1	20	20	10	10		120	3.1	3.1
7–9	350	350	32		0.1	0.1	20	20	10	10		120	2.8	2.8
10–12	350	350	32		0.1	0.1	20	20	10	10		120	2.8	2.8
Children and adults (years)														
1–2	400		50		1.0	1.0	20	20	10	10		56	4.0	3.9
3–4	400		50		1.0	1.0	20	20	10	10		44	4.0	3.9
5–6	400		102		1.0	1.0	20	20	10	10		40	4.0	3.9
7–10	400		102		1.0	1.0	20	20	2.5	2.5		40	4.0	3.9
11–12	500		102		1.0	1.0	20	20	2.5	2.5		40	7.0	6.6
13–14	600		170		1.0	1.0	30	30	2.5	2.5	34	40	7.0	6.6
15–16	600	500	170		1.0	1.0	30	30	2.5	2.5	34	40	7.0	5.5
17–18	600	500	200	170	1.0	1.0	30	30	2.5	2.5	34	40	7.0	5.5
19+	600	500	200	170	1.0	1.0	30	30	2.5	2.5	18	43	5.5	5.5
Pregnant women		600		370 to 470		1.4		50		10		[f]		6.4 to 7.5
Lactating women		850		270		1.3		50		10		24		13.7
Postmenopausal women		500		170		1.0		30		2.5		18		5.5

[a] Adapted from reference 2.
[b] Minimum level considered safe.
[c] Adapted from reference 3; 2.5 µg of cholecalciferol are equivalent to 100 IU of vitamin D.
[d] The amount of absorbed iron is a variable proportion of the intake, depending on the type of diet.
[e] Adapted from reference 4.
[f] Requirements during pregnancy depend on the woman's iron status before pregnancy.

REFERENCES

1. WHO Technical Report Series, No. 724, 1985 (*Energy and protein requirements*: report of a Joint FAO/WHO/UNU Expert Consultation).
2. FAO Food and Nutrition Series, No. 23, 1988 (*Requirements of vitamin A, iron, folate and vitamin B_{12}*: report of a Joint FAO/WHO Expert Consultation).
3. WHO Technical Report Series, No. 452, 1970 (*Requirements of ascorbic acid, vitamin D, vitamin B_{12}, folate and iron*: report of a Joint FAO/WHO Expert Group).
4. WHO Technical Report Series, No. 532, 1973 (*Trace elements in human nutrition*: report of a WHO Expert Committee).

Annex 2

DIETARY GUIDELINES FOR DIABETES MELLITUS

A number of expert groups have considered dietary recommendations for both the primary prevention and the management of diabetes mellitus. Expert groups in Europe and the USA have specified that preventing weight gain is a key to minimizing the risk of diabetes, and that even modest increases in weight in adulthood should be avoided in those who are prone to diabetes because of a family history of this condition.

Table A2.1 summarizes the dietary guidelines advocated by three expert groups. These guidelines are individual dietary recommendations and not national averages. All three expert groups emphasize the prime importance of achieving a desirable body weight and, if possible, preventing weight gain in the first place. The dietary recommendations do not differ between those with insulin-dependent diabetes and those with non-insulin-dependent diabetes. Most of the latter, however, are overweight and can produce profound changes in their condition by losing even moderate amounts of weight. There is continuing debate about whether all individuals benefit from a low-fat, high-carbohydrate diet, particularly if their blood levels of triglycerides are elevated, and some concern is expressed as to whether people used to an "affluent" diet can adjust to the major changes in diet advocated. Nevertheless, the consistency of the principal recommendations of the three groups is impressive, and the European Association for the Study of Diabetes noted that these nutritional recommendations should be applicable to all populations whatever their usual dietary habits.

Table A2.1. Recommendations on body weight, physical activity, and nutrient intakes made by North American and European expert groups concerned with the management of diabetes

	American Diabetes Association, 1986	US National Institute of Health, 1987	European Association for the Study of Diabetes, 1988
Body weight	Maintain desirable weight	Essential to maintain desirable weight as primary goal	Maintain body-mass index of 25 or reduce it to below 25 if possible
Physical activity	Aerobic regular exercise	Regular non-stressful exercise	[a]
Carbohydrate (% energy)	55–60	50–60	50–60
(a) Complex	Maximize	Beneficial for many if tolerated	Maximize
(b) Sugars	Modest only	Sucrose <5% of carbohydrate intake, i.e., <3% energy	Added sucrose <30 g/day
(c) Fibre	Maximize, e.g., 40 g of total fibre/1000 $kcal_{th}$ or 25 g of non-starch polysaccharides/1000 $kcal_{th}$	Potential benefits	Maximize soluble fibre: up to 20 g/1000 $kcal_{th}$
Total fat (% energy)	<30	<30	<30
Saturated fatty acids (% energy)	Reduce to <10	<10	<10
Polyunsaturated fatty acids	Some substitution for saturated fats possible; 6–8% energy	[a]	Equal intakes of mono- and polyunsaturated fatty acids
Dietary cholesterol (mg/day)	<300	[a]	<300
Alcohol	Moderate	[a]	Moderate: only with meals. Avoid if overweight or hypertensive, or if blood lipid levels are high
Sodium	<1 g/1000 $kcal_{th}$; maximum 3 g/day	[a]	Restrict to <6 g/day; if hypertensive <3 g/day
Protein	Normal RDA 0.8 g/kg of body weight	12–20% energy	Avoid high intakes

[a] No recommendation made.

172

GOLDEN RULES FOR SAFE FOOD PREPARATION

Illness due to contaminated food is a widespread health problem; in infants and the elderly, its consequences can be fatal. WHO data indicate that only a small number of factors are responsible for a large proportion of foodborne disease episodes. Common errors include:

- preparation of food too far ahead of consumption
- prepared food being left too long at a temperature that permits bacterial proliferation
- inadequate heating
- cross-contamination
- an infected or "colonized" person handling the food.

The Ten Golden Rules presented below respond to these errors, offering advice that can reduce the risk that foodborne pathogens will be able to contaminate, to survive, or to multiply. The rules have been drawn up by the World Health Organization to provide guidance to members of the community on safe food preparation in the home. They should be adapted, as appropriate, to local conditions.

1. Choose foods processed for safety

While many foods, such as fruits and vegetables, are best in their natural state, others simply are not safe unless they have been processed. For example, always buy pasteurized as opposed to raw milk and, if you have the choice, select fresh or frozen poultry treated with ionizing radiation. When shopping, keep in mind that food processing was invented to improve safety as well as to prolong shelf-life. Certain foods eaten raw, such as lettuce, need thorough washing.

2. Cook food thoroughly

Many raw foods, most notably poultry, meats, and unpasteurized milk, are very often contaminated with disease-causing pathogens. Thorough cooking will kill the pathogens, but remember that the temperature of *all parts of the food* must reach at least 70 °C. If cooked chicken is still raw near the bone, put it back in the oven until it is done—all the way through. Frozen meat, fish, and poultry must be thoroughly thawed *before* cooking.

3. Eat cooked foods immediately

When cooked foods cool to room temperature, microbes begin to proliferate. The longer the wait, the greater the risk. To be on the safe side, eat cooked foods as soon as they come off the heat.

4. Store cooked foods carefully

If you must prepare foods in advance or want to keep leftovers, be sure to store them under either hot (near or above 60 °C) or cool (near or below 10 °C) conditions. This rule is of vital importance if you plan to store foods for more than four or five hours. *Foods for infants should preferably not be stored at all.* A common error, responsible for countless cases of foodborne disease, is to put too large a quantity of warm food in the refrigerator. In an over-burdened refrigerator, cooked foods cannot cool to the core as quickly as they must. When the centre of food remains warm (above 10 °C) too long, microbes thrive, quickly proliferating to disease-producing levels.

5. Reheat cooked foods thoroughly

This is your best protection against microbes that may have developed during storage (proper storage slows down microbial growth but does not kill the organisms). Once again, thorough reheating means that *all parts of the food* must reach at least 70 °C.

6. Avoid contact between raw foods and cooked foods

Safely cooked food can become contaminated through even the slightest contact with raw food. This cross-contamination can be direct, as when raw poultry meat comes into contact with cooked foods. It can also be more subtle. For example, do not prepare a raw chicken and then use the same unwashed cutting board and knife to carve the cooked bird. Doing so can reintroduce all the potential risks for microbial growth and subsequent illness present prior to cooking.

174

7. Wash hands repeatedly

Wash hands thoroughly before you start preparing food and after every interruption—especially if you have to change the baby or have been to the toilet. After preparing raw foods such as fish, meat, or poultry, wash again before you start handling other foods. And if you have an infection on your hand, be sure to bandage or cover it before preparing food. Remember, too, that household pets—dogs, birds, and especially turtles—often harbour dangerous pathogens that can pass from your hands into food.

8. Keep all kitchen surfaces meticulously clean

Since foods are easily contaminated, any surface used for food preparation must be kept absolutely clean. Think of every food scrap, crumb or spot as a potential reservoir of germs. Cloths that come into contact with dishes and utensils should be changed every day and boiled before reuse. Separate cloths for cleaning the floors also require frequent washing.

9. Protect foods from insects, rodents, and other animals

Animals frequently carry pathogenic microorganisms which cause foodborne disease. Storing foods in tightly sealed containers is your best protection.

10. Use pure water

Pure water is just as important for food preparation as for drinking. If you have any doubts about the water supply, boil water before adding it to food or making ice for drinks. Be especially careful with any water used to prepare an infant's meal.

Annex 4

A REVIEW OF DIETARY RECOMMENDATIONS IN DEVELOPED AND DEVELOPING COUNTRIES[1]

Official recommendations for overall health maintenance issued by government agencies in different countries, or by various expert panels, are summarized in Table A4.1 (pages 180–181).

Table A4.2 (pages 182–183) summarizes various proposed dietary recommendations aimed at lowering the risk of cardiovascular diseases in the general population and/or high-risk groups.

Dietary guidelines that have been proposed with the object of lowering cancer risk are summarized in Table A4.3 (pages 184–185).

REFERENCES

1. COMMONWEALTH DEPARTMENT OF HEALTH. *Nutrition policy statements*. Canberra, Australian Government Publishing Service, 1984.
2. COMMONWEALTH DEPARTMENT OF HEALTH. *Towards better nutrition for Australians. Report of the Nutrition Task Force of the Better Health Commission.* Canberra, Australian Government Publishing Service, 1987.
3. DEPARTMENT OF NATIONAL HEALTH AND WELFARE. *Canada's food guide handbook (revised)*. Ontario, Ottawa Supply and Services, 1982.
4. HEJDA, S. & OSANCOVA, K. *Dietary guidelines for the population [Czechoslovakia]*. Society for Rational Nutrition. Presented at the International Conference on Dietary Guidelines, 27–28 June 1988. Ryerson Polytechnic Institute, Toronto, Canada.
5. DUPIN, H. ET AL. *Apports nutritionnels conseillés pour la population française,* 3rd ed. [*Recommended nutritional intakes for the French population.*] Paris, Technique et Documentation Lavoisier, 1981.
6. GERMAN SOCIETY OF NUTRITION. *Ten guidelines for sensible nutrition*. Frankfurt, Deutsche Gesellschaft für Ernährung, 1985.
7. COMPLEX COMMITTEE ON FOOD SCIENCE OF THE HUNGARIAN ACADEMY OF SCIENCES AND OF THE MINISTRY OF FOOD AND AGRICULTURE, NATIONAL INSTITUTE OF FOOD HYGIENE AND NUTRITION, AND HUNGARIAN SOCIETY FOR NUTRITION. [Dietary guidelines for Hungarians.] Budapest, 1988 (In Hungarian).
8. GOPALAN, C. *Dietary guidelines from the perspective of developing countries*. Presented at the International Conference on Dietary Guidelines, 27–28 June, 1988. Ryerson Polytechnic Institute, Toronto.
9. FOOD ADVISORY COMMITTEE OF THE IRISH DEPARTMENT OF HEALTH. *Guidelines for preparing information and advice to the general public on healthy eating habits.* Dublin, Department of Health, 1984.

---

[1] All the tables in this Annex were prepared by Dr S. Palmer, based on material collected for: NATIONAL RESEARCH COUNCIL. *Diet and health: implications for reducing chronic disease risk*. Washington, DC, National Academy Press, 1989.

10. MINISTRY OF HEALTH AND WELFARE. *Dietary guidelines for health promotion,* Vol. 29. Tokyo, Health Promotion and Nutrition Division, Health Services Bureau, Ministry of Health and Welfare, 1985 (*The nutrition of Japan,* **20**(4): 29–172 to 29–177).

11. BENGOA, J.M. ET AL. *Guias de alimentación—bases para su desarrollo en América Latina* [Alimentary guidelines—bases for their development in Latin America.] Venezuela, United Nations University and Fundación Cavendes, 1988.

12. FOOD AND NUTRITION COUNCIL. *Nota voedingsbeleid. [Food policy note.]* The Hague, Ministry of Health, Welfare, and Culture; Ministry of Agriculture; and the Ministry of Economics, 1983–84.

13. THE NUTRITION BOARD. Guidelines for healthy food. Condensed from the recommendations of the Nutrition Board. *The Netherlands journal of nutrition,* **47**(5): 140–142 (1986).

14. NUTRITION ADVISORY COMMITTEE. Nutrition goals for New Zealanders. *Quarterly magazine of New Zealand Department of Health,* **34**: 11–12 (1982).

15. ROYAL MINISTRY OF HEALTH AND SOCIAL AFFAIRS. *Report No. 11 to the Storting: on the follow-up of Norwegian nutrition policy.* Oslo, 1981–82.

16. BERGER, S. *Dietary guidelines in Eastern European countries.* Presented at the International Conference on Dietary Guidelines, 27–28 June 1988. Ryerson Polytechnic Institute, Toronto, Canada.

17. *Swedish nutrition recommendation.* Uppsala, The National Food Administration, 1981.

18. SWEDISH EXPERT GROUP FOR DIET AND HEALTH. *A summary of the report from the Expert Group for Diet and Health.* Uppsala, The Food Committee of 1983, 1985.

19. NATIONAL ADVISORY COMMITTEE FOR NUTRITION EDUCATION. *A discussion paper on proposals for nutritional guidelines for health education in Britain.* London, Health Education Council, 1983.

20. US CONGRESS. *Dietary goals for the United States,* 2nd ed. *Report of the Select Committee on Nutrition and Human Needs.* Washington, DC, US Government Printing Office, 1977 (Stock No. 052-070-04376-8).

21. OFFICE OF THE ASSISTANT SECRETARY FOR HEALTH AND SURGEON GENERAL, PUBLIC HEALTH SERVICE, US DEPARTMENT OF HEALTH, EDUCATION AND WELFARE. *Healthy people: the Surgeon General's report on health promotion and disease prevention.* Washington, DC, US Government Printing Office, 1979 (DHEW (PHS) Publ. No. 79-55071).

22. US DEPARTMENT OF AGRICULTURE/DEPARTMENT OF HEALTH AND HUMAN SERVICES. *Nutrition and your health: dietary guidelines for Americans,* 2nd ed. Washington, DC, US Government Printing Office, 1985 (Home and garden bulletin No. 232).

23. US DEPARTMENT OF HEALTH AND HUMAN SERVICES, PUBLIC HEALTH SERVICE. *The Surgeon General's report on nutrition and health.* Washington, DC, US Government Printing Office, 1988 (DHHS (PHS) Publ. No. 88-50210).

24. NATIONAL RESEARCH COUNCIL. *Diet and health: implications for reducing chronic disease risk.* Washington, DC, National Academy Press, 1989.

25. JAMES, W.P.T. ET AL. *Healthy nutrition: preventing nutrition-related diseases in Europe.* Copenhagen, WHO Regional Office for Europe, 1988 (WHO Regional Publications, European Series, No. 24).

26. COMMITTEE OF DIET AND HEART DISEASE OF THE NATIONAL HEART FOUNDATION OF AUSTRALIA. Diet and coronary heart disease: a review. *Medical journal of Australia,* **2**: 294–307 (1979).

27. DEPARTMENT OF NATIONAL HEALTH AND WELFARE. *Recommendations for prevention programs in relation to nutrition and cardiovascular disease.* Ottawa, Bureau of Nutritional Sciences, Health Protection Branch, 1977.

28. *Preliminary report of the Canadian Consensus Conference on Cholesterol. A conference on the prevention of heart and vascular disease through altering serum lipid and lipoprotein risk factors, Ottawa, 9–11 March 1988.* Ottawa, The Government Conference Centre, 1988.

29. EUROPEAN ATHEROSCLEROSIS SOCIETY STUDY GROUP. Strategies for the prevention of coronary heart disease: a policy statement of the European Atherosclerosis Society. *European heart journal,* **8**: 77–88 (1987).

30. FINNISH HEART ASSOCIATION, NATIONAL BOARD OF HEALTH, NATIONAL PUBLIC HEALTH INSTITUTE, AND FINNISH CARDIAC SOCIETY. *Prevention of coronary heart disease in Finland.* Helsinki, Finnish Heart Association, 1987.

31. Official recommendations on diet in the Scandinavian countries. *Nutrition reviews,* **26**: 259–263 (1968).

32. Dietary fat and degenerative vascular diseases. *Nutrition and metabolism,* **18**: 113–115 (1975).

33. PUBLIC HEALTH BUREAU AND THE JAPANESE DIETETIC ASSOCIATION PANEL ON NUTRITION AND PREVENTION OF DISEASES. *Dietary guidelines and nutrition policies in Japan.* Tokyo, Ministry of Health and Welfare, 1983.

34. NETHERLANDS NUTRITION COUNCIL. Recommendation on amount and nature of dietary fats. *Voeding,* **34**: 552–557 (1973).

35. NATIONAL HEART FOUNDATION OF NEW ZEALAND. *Coronary heart disease. A progress report.* Dunedin, New Zealand, John McIndoe Ltd. and National Heart Foundation of New Zealand, 1976.

36. AD HOC WORKING GROUP ON CORONARY PREVENTION. Prevention of coronary heart disease in the United Kingdom. *Lancet,* **i**: 846–847 (1982).

37. DEPARTMENT OF HEALTH AND SOCIAL SECURITY/COMMITTEE ON MEDICAL ASPECTS OF FOOD POLICY. *Diet and cardiovascular disease. Report of the Panel on Diet in Relation to Cardiovascular Disease.* London, Her Majesty's Stationery Office, 1984 (Report on Health and Social Subjects No. 28).

38. INTER-SOCIETY COMMISSION FOR HEART DISEASE RESOURCES. Optimal resources for primary prevention of atherosclerotic diseases. *Circulation,* **70**: 153A–205A (1984).

39. NATIONAL INSTITUTES OF HEALTH. Lowering blood cholesterol to prevent heart disease. *Journal of the American Medical Association,* **253**: 2080–2086 (1985).

40. GRUNDY, S.M. ET AL. Rationale of the diet-health statement of the American Heart Association. Report of Nutrition Committee. *Circulation,* **65**: 839A–854A (1982).

41. AMERICAN HEART ASSOCIATION. Dietary guidelines for healthy American adults: a statement for physicians and health professionals by the Nutrition Committee, American Heart Association. *Circulation,* **77**: 721A–724A (1988).

42. WHO Technical Report Series, No. 678, 1982 (*Prevention of coronary heart disease*: report of a WHO Expert Committee).

43. CANADIAN CANCER SOCIETY. *Facts on cancer and diet. Your food choices may help you reduce your cancer risk.* Toronto, Canadian Cancer Society, 1985.

44. Report of the joint ECP-IUNS workshop on diet and human carcinogenesis, Aarhus (Denmark), 17–19 June 1985. In: Joossens, J.V. et al., ed. *Diet and human carcinogenesis.* Amsterdam, Excerpta Medica, 1985, pp. 335–342.

45. COMMITTEE ON DIET, NUTRITION AND CANCER, ASSEMBLY OF LIFE SCIENCES, NATIONAL RESEARCH COUNCIL. *Diet, nutrition, and cancer.* Washington, DC, National Academy Press, 1982.
46. AMERICAN CANCER SOCIETY. *Nutrition and cancer: cause and prevention. American Cancer Society Special Report.* New York, American Cancer Society, 1984.
47. NATIONAL CANCER INSTITUTE, NATIONAL INSTITUTES OF HEALTH. *Diet, nutrition, and cancer prevention: a guide to food choices.* Washington, DC, US Government Printing Office, 1987 (NIH Publ. No. 87-2878).

Table A4.1. Dietary recommendations in industrialized and developing countries, 197

Country/region or source of recommendation	Annex 4 reference No.	Target group(s)	Maintain appropriate body weight, exercise	Limit or reduce total fat (% energy)	Reduce saturated fatt acids (% energy)
Australia 1983	1	GP	Yes	Yes	NC
1987, targets for 1995	2	GP	Reduce obesity prevalence to 30%	35%	NS
1987, targets for 2000	2	GP	To 25%	33%	NS
Canada 1982	3	GP	Yes	35%	Yes
Czechoslovakia 1988	4	GP	Yes, reduce by 10–15%	Yes, reduce by 15 g/day	Yes
France 1981	5	GP	Yes	30–35%	Yes
Germany, Federal Republic of, 1985	6	GP	Yes	Yes	NS
Hungary 1988	7	GP	Yes	Avoid too much	Use vegetable oil
India 1988	8	HR (affluent people)	Yes	15–20%	NC
Ireland 1984	9	GP	Yes	≤35%	Yes
Japan 1985	10	GP	Yes	20–25%	Yes
Latin America 1988	11	GP	Yes	20–25%	≤8
Netherlands 1983–1984	12	GP	Yes	30–35%	Yes
1986	13	GP	Yes	30–35%	Yes
New Zealand 1982	14	GP HR	Yes	Yes	Yes
Norway 1981–1982	15	GP	NC	<35%	Yes
Poland 1988	16	GP	Yes	≈30%	Yes
Sweden 1981	17	GP	Yes	25–35%	Yes
1985	18	GP	Yes	Reduce by 5% energy by 1990; to ≈30% by 2000	NS
United Kingdom 1983	19	GP	Yes	30%	10
United States of America 1977	20	GP	Yes	27–33%	Yes
1979	21	GP	Yes	Yes	Yes
1985	22	GP	Yes	Yes	Yes
1988	23	GP HR	Yes	Yes	Yes
1989	24	GP	Balance energy intake and expenditure	≤30%	<10% for individuals 7–8% population mean
WHO 1988 Intermediate goals	25	GP	BMI	35%	15%
Ultimate goals			20–25	20–30%	10–15%

[a] BMI = body-mass index; GP = General population; HR = High-risk groups; NC = No comment; NS = Not specified; P/S = Ratio of po

Sodium chloride (g/day)	Alcohol intake	Other recommendations
Restrict	Moderation	Focus on HR groups; food labelling; recommendations safe for GP
Restrict	NC	Variety of foods
Limit	Limit	Focus on HR groups; limit protein to 10–15% energy
Moderation	Moderation, <25–30 g/day	Nutrition education; collaboration among government and other groups; food labelling
Reduce; for HR <5	Moderation	Avoid trace element deficiencies; food labelling; focus on HR groups
NC	NC	10–12% of energy from protein; 30–50% of animal origin
NC	NC	NC
Limit to <10	Avoid too much	Variety; eat enough protein, half from vegetables and half from animal sources; eat enough potassium, especially from green vegetables; eat lean meat and fish and fewer sweets
NC	NC	NC
NC	Restrict to reduce weight	NC
NC	NC	Special attention to children
Decrease	Avoid excess; <90 ml/day males; <65 ml/day females	Special recommendations for governments, professionals, industry
5	NC	NC
NC	NC	Guidelines for health professionals, industry, and public
<3 (as sodium)	30–50 g ethanol/day	Protein to make up remainder of energy; wide variety of foods
<5	Drink less	Emphasis on plant foods, fish, poultry, lean meats, low-fat dairy products and fewer whole eggs
<5	Limit	Increase nutrient density; water fluoridation 0.7–1.2 mg/l; iodine prophylaxis; intermediate and ultimate goals

Table A4.3. Dietary recommendations to reduce cancer risk in industrialized countrie

Country/region	Annex 4 reference No.	Maintain appropriate body weight, exercise	Limit or reduce total fat (% energy)	Modify ratio of dietary fats	Promote fruit and vegetable intake	Increase complex carbohyd fibre inta
Canada 1985	43	Yes	Reduce	Decrase saturated fatty acids and cholesterol	Yes	More fibe containin foods
Europe 1986	44	Yes	To ≈30	NC	Yes	Yes
Japan 1983	33	NC	Avoid excess	NC	Especially green/yellow vegetables, oranges, carotene, and fungi	Unrefine cereal, seafood, fibre-rich legumes
United States of America 1982	45	NC	To ≈30	NC	Especially citrus fruits, green and yellow and cruciferous vegetables	Whole-gr products vegetabl and fruits
1984	46	Yes	To ≈30	NC	Especially vitamin A- and C-rich foods and cruciferous vegetables	High-fibr foods, w grain cer
1987	47	Yes	To ≈30	NC	Vitamin A-rich, green and yellow vegetables, citrus fruits	Whole-gr products, 20–30 g fibre/day

[a] NC = No comment; NS = Not specified.

Restrict sodium chloride	Food preparation methods	Alcohol intake	Other recommendations
NS	Minimize cured, pickled, and smoked foods	Two or fewer drinks per day, if any	NC
To <5 g/day	As above; avoid frying and high-temperature cooking	Drink less, if at all	Varied diet; no food supplements; recommendations to government, scientists, and industry
Yes	Avoid hot drinks and burned food	Drink less, if at all	Varied diet; chew food well
Minimize cured and pickled foods	Minimize cured, pickled, and smoked foods	Drink less, if at all	Avoid food supplements; monitor and test mutagens and carcinogens; recommendations to government, scientists and industry
NS	As above	As above	NC
NS	As above; avoid frying and high-temperature cooking	As above	Balanced diet; read labels; follow guidelines given in reference 3

TECHNICAL CONSIDERATIONS CONCERNING IMPLEMENTATION OF RECOMMENDATIONS AT THE NATIONAL LEVEL

Introduction

Nutrient goals must be set and the existing nutrient intakes of the population must be known before a start can be made in developing national policies and actions relating to the modification of dietary intakes in order to reduce the population risk of chronic diseases. The patterns of food use that determine the nutrient intakes must also be understood so that targets for nutrient change can be translated into targets for dietary change, or dietary intake goals.

Implementation assumes not only an overall policy decision to include nutritional goals as a part of health, agriculture, and economic policies, but also the technical resources to translate the policy into appropriate guidelines for modifying food use and nutrient intake. Effective implementation also requires a surveillance system to monitor the process, so that the programme can be progressively adjusted.

The following paragraphs are intended to clarify concepts in the main report relating to the interpretation and application of nutrient goals. The comments are directed primarily to those providing technical back-up for policy-makers and programme designers. The purpose is to highlight the differences from previous approaches, rather than to provide explicit guidance on interpretation. Additional information can be obtained from the list of publications at the end of this annex.

Nutrition surveillance systems: impact of present recommendations

During the past decade, several United Nations agencies and bilateral donors have worked with the governments of developing countries to develop and implement nutrition surveillance programmes. Surveillance, in this connotation, must be explicitly differentiated from the older concept of "surveys". Explicitly, "surveillance" refers to the collection and use of data as part of current planning and implementation activities. The type of data to be collected, as well as the methods used, must be appropriate to ensure that the surveillance process can be used by those responsible for developing and implementing the policy and programme. Surveillance is more concerned with the use of data, and hence with the definition of data needed by the user, than with the collection of information (1, 2, 3). The surveillance activities undertaken so far in developing countries have placed great emphasis on the surveillance of problems related to undernutrition. Surveillance systems focusing on the problems of overnutrition have only begun to emerge in industrialized countries in recent years (4).

It is clear that surveillance systems in developing countries should now take into account both undernutrition and overnutrition. This recommendation calls for an expansion of the scope of activities rather than a radical modification of the principles or design of surveillance.

Present systems designed to monitor those at risk of nutrient deficiency (e.g., the more impoverished sectors of societies) should now evolve to include nutrient surveillance of the more privileged sectors, using different assessment techniques where necessary. In developing countries, where major disparities in diets and effective access to food and health care are a problem, an analysis of national per caput dietary data may not be very meaningful. Disaggregated information on the distribution of intakes in specific groups, defined in social or economic terms, may be more appropriate than concentrating only on vulnerable groups, e.g., children, pregnant women, and the elderly. Thus, for example, it may be important to monitor, differentially, the trends in intake and in disease patterns in the subsistence farming community, in the periurban and urban poor, in the urban middle class, and in the privileged groups. In some societies, it is possible to find opposite gradients in problems of undernutrition and overnutrition in the rural and urban areas, according to the degree of affluence. It will often be equally important to engage in some long-term activities, for example in education, among sectors of the population in which current food-usage patterns are very different from those expected in the future. Nevertheless, the long-term strategy should be to establish sound dietary practices in all sectors of the population, for the prevention of both undernutrition and overnutrition. The planner must recognize that in a single country or region there may be such a diversity of food patterns that to achieve the same set of nutritional goals, the dietary habits of the extreme subgroups of society may have to move in opposite directions.

The "population approach" espoused in this report does not imply that such differentiation of sectors should be avoided. Rather, it argues that where meaningful subpopulation differentiations can be made, they are to be encouraged. In contrast, the "population approach" specifically argues against differentiation down to the level of the individual. It adopts the position that a national goal must involve the modification and improvement of the environment in which individuals make their choices, as well as improve the ability of the individuals to make wise choices. This philosophy is gaining wide acceptance in many countries (5). It must be recognized also that a single population nutrient goal does not imply conformity in food-use practices; there is ample room for individual variation. The goal should be that individual differences in food selection provide a distribution centred on the stipulated population nutrient goal, and not that dietary prescriptions are imposed on the individual.

Dietary monitoring: baseline information and trend analysis

In section 5 of the main report, the difference between population goals and recommended intakes applied to individuals was made clear. This was further illustrated in Fig. 18 (page 118). Since technical staff involved in the assessment of dietary conditions will be concerned both with the current population nutrient goals (expressed as mean nutrient concentrations or mean intakes) and with estimates of nutrient requirements of individuals previously published by FAO/WHO committees, the following paragraphs again direct attention to the distinction, and to the implications for application.

Population nutrient goals

Conceptually, population nutrient goals relate to the mean intake of the total population, the intakes of all ages and sexes being taken as a single distribution. For protein, carbohydrate, fat, and the different classes of fatty acids, these have been expressed as nutrient concentrations or nutrient:energy ratios (percentage of total energy). In the paragraphs above, it has been noted that, for assessment and planning purposes, the population may be subdivided into subpopulation groups. The goals expressed in relation to energy intake are thought to be age and sex insensitive.[1] That is, no adjustment is needed to take into account different demographic profiles of the subpopulation groups. In the case of salt and cholesterol intake, the goals were expressed as absolute intakes per day, again referring to a population or subpopulation mean. These estimates are sensitive to both age and sex. If there is a major difference in demographic profile between the subpopulation groups, some adjustment of goals would be appropriate. It is suggested that it be assumed that the appropriate goal would be proportional to total food intake, measured as energy intake. Approaches to the estimation of population per caput energy needs, based on the estimates of an FAO/WHO/UNU expert consultation (6), have been described by James & Schofield (7). The subpopulation goal would be appropriately seen as shown below.

Goal for subpopulation mean nutrient intake =

$$\frac{\text{Population nutrient goal}}{\text{Population per caput energy need}} \times \begin{array}{c} \text{Subpopulation mean} \\ \text{energy intake} \end{array}$$

Since this approach takes into account, in an empirical manner, the demographic composition of the subpopulation, no further adjustment is needed. The obvious limitation is that it reflects existing energy intakes rather than desirable levels of intakes; for longer-term goals, it may be necessary to adjust the subpopulation goals as both demography changes and energy intakes approach desirable levels. If energy-intake data are available for only some demographic strata of the subpopulation, an adjusted goal for those strata can be derived.

In the initial assessment, the position of the population or subpopulation mean relative to the goal must be ascertained. The magnitude of the difference between the two will determine the magnitude of shift in the population distribution that is desired. There will be interest in examining the distribution of intakes within populations and subpopulation groups for suggestions of other

---

[1] Goals expressed as proportion of energy are therefore applicable to all age and sex groups after early childhood. In the case of goals expressed as absolute intakes, actual intakes would be expected to be proportional to total food intake; thus, children would be expected to consume less salt or cholesterol than adults, and women less than men.

distinctive subgroups. There should be no attempt to assess individual intakes in relation to the population nutrient goals (see section 5).

In trend analysis, the objective is to monitor progress of the population or subpopulation mean intakes towards the population goal. If sample surveys, or sentinel population surveys, are used to collect data, care should be taken to ensure that sampling differences do not seriously distort the trend picture.

Undoubtedly, there will be interest in monitoring the per caput food "disappearance" data, as assembled by national governments, or by FAO on their behalf. Two cautions are needed. First, in a country confronted with both inadequacies and excesses of dietary intakes, the per caput figures may be misleading. Second, disappearance data, although often expressed as "per caput intake" may often overestimate actual intakes (8). Further, since the proportional overestimation may differ between energy sources, it is not necessarily true that the estimate of a nutrient in terms of a percentage of energy will be the same in the disappearance data as it would be in nutrient intake data. Wherever possible, technical personnel at the country level should attempt to validate per caput disappearance data against intake data (e.g., where a national sample survey has been conducted, the nutrient:energy ratios determined for per caput disappearance data and survey data may be compared). Provided that the magnitude of any bias can be estimated, and account is taken of the difficulties that arise when distribution within the population is very uneven, per caput food disappearance data can be a very useful adjunct in trend monitoring and surveillance.

"Recommended" or "safe" levels of nutrient intake

As noted in section 5, previous FAO/WHO reports on nutrient requirements have addressed the distribution of requirements among similar individuals, e.g., among adult men, adult women, children, or specified ages and sexes (see also Annex 1 to this report). The goal has been to define the level of intake that is sufficiently high to meet the needs of almost all individuals, including those with the upper range of requirements. (The exception is energy, where previous reports have explicitly addressed the average requirement of a group of comparable individuals). The approach to application and interpretation of the estimates of nutrient requirements of

190

individuals is very different from that described in the present report for the population nutrient goals. This difference must be taken into account by surveillance staff, who will be concerned with monitoring both the nutrients discussed in the present report and those discussed in previous reports (e.g., iron, vitamin A, and vitamin C).

When the distributions of individual needs have been estimated, the appropriate approach to assessment of observed intakes is the "probability assessment" in which the likelihood of inadequacy is assessed on the basis of the relative position of the observed intake within the estimated distribution of requirements. This approach has evolved through a series of FAO/WHO reports (6, 9, 10). Recently this approach and its application to observed distributions of intakes have been examined in detail and the concept has been validated by a committee in the USA (11). That committee's report also addressed approaches to eliminating the bias in the estimated prevalence of inadequate intakes introduced by day-to-day variation in intakes (see also 12).

Distributions of nutrient requirements have been estimated for relatively homogeneous groups of individuals. In some cases, serious problems can arise when attempts are made to pool these estimates as in the derivation of population estimates. A notable example of the interpretational difficulties is found with iron. Iron intakes are not distributed in proportion to need, since women have much higher needs than men but consume smaller amounts of food and hence of iron (there is little characteristic difference in the mix of foods, and hence iron concentrations, consumed by men and women). A per caput intake that appears to be adequate on the basis of pooled requirement estimates might therefore represent higher than necessary intakes for men and inadequate intakes for many women (13). Other distributional considerations make it very difficult to develop per caput requirement estimates for the micronutrients, although it is theoretically possible to do so for demographic strata in subpopulation groups in which it is thought that distributions are not distorted by major inequities. For the micronutrients, and where survey data are available, it is recommended that technical staff apply the probability approach discussed in the references cited above. Here, baseline data would be expressed in terms of the estimated prevalence of inadequate intakes, and trend analyses might relate to changes both in this prevalence and in the population mean intakes (without defined goals for the latter).

Nutrient density ratios for micronutrients

Theoretically, expression of micronutrient requirements in relation to energy needs (e.g., nutrient per 1000 kcal$_{th}$) might overcome some of the problems of differences in intake and in requirement across age and sex strata. This would be true where the nutrient requirement and energy requirement change in parallel across such strata (but would not be true for iron, as indicated above). In the past, some have calculated a reference nutrient:energy ratio as the ratio of the "recommended intake" of the nutrient divided by the average energy requirement, multiplied by 1000. This is an incorrect procedure if the derived ratio is intended to have the same meaning as the recommended intake. A correct approach to deriving the ratio, applicable to individuals, and taking into account the bivariate distribution of both nutrient and energy requirements, was described in the report by the Joint FAO/WHO/UNU Expert Consultation on energy and protein requirements (6). That report pointed out that, for application to population data, it would be necessary also to take into account the expected variation of nutrient:energy ratios in the population (see also 14). Energy ratios would still be applicable to population data stratified by age, sex, and physiological status. The theoretical basis and statistical approaches for derivation of reference nutrient:energy ratios, comparable in intent to the population nutrient goals, have been developed. The ratios have not been generally published and their utility has not been fully tested. Those wishing to attempt to develop a set of nutrient density goals for application in planning and surveillance might wish to consult the references cited.

Outcome monitoring

The stated objective of a nutrition surveillance programme, and of the population nutrient goals discussed in this report, is the encouragement of dietary intakes compatible with minimal rates of morbidity and preventable mortality. An obvious approach to monitoring implementation is the examination of trends in these disease patterns. To target educational or other intervention programmes, it is necessary to examine the distribution of outcomes in the population, disaggregated into subpopulation groups as discussed above. In the present report, chronic diseases are the focus of attention. Morbidity, mortality, and anthropometric indicators of obesity are the outcomes of interest. Seldom are morbidity data (or blood pressure data) available without special sample surveys. Mortality data, however, are customarily collected and should be disaggregated, if possible, according to age, sex, disease, etc. Due note must be taken of the expected lag between change in dietary intake and the manifestation of an associated change in mortality, since it is assumed that diet influences the long-term development of the conditions involved. In the specific case of obesity, it is recommended that existing surveillance systems, designed to collect anthropometric data for children, be expanded to include adults, and that obesity as well as undersize and thinness be reported.

For the deficiency diseases, much has been written already with regard to approaches to the collection and interpretation of data on outcome (e.g., xerophthalmia as a manifestation of vitamin A deficiency; goitre as a manifestation of iodine deficiency; anaemia as a manifestation of iron, folate, or vitamin B_{12} deficiency).

Although some form of baseline dietary information is needed for planning purposes, and periodic updating of this information is required in monitoring and surveillance, it may be easier and more effective, for surveillance purposes, to focus on indicators of nutritional status. Thus, for example, it may be more effective to monitor serum retinol levels in a population than to collect information about dietary vitamin A intakes. In the specific cases of iodine and sodium (salt), dietary studies are probably inadequate for the estimation of total intake. In these two instances, better estimates can be obtained by measuring urinary excretion, taking into account losses by other routes. Certainly, in any surveillance programme covering salt intake and hypertension, monitoring urinary sodium levels is a preferred approach.

Relation to existing nutrition programmes

The present report has emphasized a population approach to the control of diet-related chronic diseases, and the reasons for this approach were presented in section 5. However, it must be recognized that in the presence of problems of inadequate intake of specific nutrients and a skewed distribution of effective demand within the population, much has been learned about the effectiveness of targeted approaches to control—activities directed towards population segments with a particularly high prevalence of the particular problem(s). This approach also recognizes that the etiology of the problem(s), and the specific opportunities for intervention, differ among the sectors of the population. Thus, for example, major distinctions must be made between the problems of (and possible approaches to) the urban poor and the rural subsistence farmer in developing countries. The recommended approach recognizes that the deficiency diseases, like the diseases associated with excessive intake, are multifactorial and that, for effective long-term control, multifaceted approaches are required (e.g., the modification of other risk factors, such as poor sanitation and inadequate primary health care). At the same time, for some of the deficiency diseases, specific short-term approaches to control can be, and are being, developed and implemented. Two specific examples are the interagency programmes for the control of blindness due to vitamin A deficiency and for the control of goitre, cretinism, and deaf-mutism due to iodine deficiency. Iron, or iron and folate, supplementation during pregnancy, and targeted food supplementation for children, in association with growth-monitoring programmes, are other examples. The "differential diagnosis" of the problem is now recognized as an important integral part of nutrition planning and of nutrition surveillance in developing countries.

Nothing in this report should be taken as arguing against this disaggregated and targeted approach to the control of nutritional deficiency diseases. Indeed, as previously noted, in some regards this experience provides a model for aspects of the control of chronic diseases where they are clustered in definable sectors of the population. These diseases are multifactorial, and are associated with environmental and life-style risk factors that are amenable to modification. In so far as these risks tend to cluster in definable population groups, there is a rationale for targeted as well as generalized population approaches. Certain principles apply to the control of problems of both inadequate and excessive nutrient intake. However, there are also major differences in the type of activities, and in the appropriate organizational structures for control. These issues must be addressed, and solutions developed, in a national context.

The Study Group recognizes the differences in the dominant nutritional problems of developed and developing countries and urges that long-term nutrition planning should strive to maintain national populations in a position where the prevalence of diseases associated with both inadequate and excessive intakes will be held to the feasible minimum.

Life-cycle considerations

The body of the present report, specifically including the sections addressing the development and application of the population nutrient goals, has focused upon the whole population, without major reference to specific age or sex groups. (It was noted nevertheless that special concerns about low fat intake, and hence low energy density of consumed diets, would apply to young children). This is appropriate for those goals, since one of the objectives is to address the overall food supply of the population or subpopulation, rather than problems related to its distribution among individuals. However, in keeping with remarks made in the preceding paragraphs, it is both appropriate and necessary for the purposes of nutrition programmes to differentiate not only the socio-demographic and environmental setting of the problems, but also the social and physiological considerations of different age and sex groups. There is now wide acceptance of the concept that activities directed towards health during pregnancy and lactation, and towards the prevention of early growth failure, represent an investment in human capital. Nutrition programmes directed towards the control of diet-related chronic disease also represent an investment in human capital through the prevention of premature mortality and disability, as well as an investment that will, in the long-term, reduce the present (developed countries) or prospective (developing countries) costs of health care. All of the evidence available suggests that, for cardiovascular diseases and for cancer, diet has an influence throughout the life cycle, even though the end-points are manifested in the adult. Thus, policies and programmes directed towards the control of nutritional inadequacies and nutritional excesses in populations throughout the world must take into account general requirements throughout the life cycle as well as the specific needs of certain groups.

References

1. WHO Technical Report Series, No. 593, 1976 (*Methodology of nutritional surveillance*: twenty-seventh report of a Joint FAO/UNICEF/WHO Expert Committee).
2. MASON, J.B. ET AL. *Nutritional surveillance*. Geneva, World Health Organization, 1984.
3. MASON, J.B. & MITCHELL, J. Nutritional surveillance. *Bulletin of the World Health Organization*, **61**: 745–755 (1983).

4. KELLY, A. *Nutritional surveillance in Europe: a critical appraisal.* Wageningen, Agricultural University, 1987 (EURO-NUT Report No. 9).
5. EPP, J. *Achieving health for all: a framework for health promotion.* Montreal, Health and Welfare, Canada, 1986.
6. WHO Technical Report Series, No. 724, 1985 (*Energy and protein requirements*: report of a Joint FAO/WHO/UNU Expert Consultation).
7. JAMES, W.P.T. & SCHOFIELD. E.C. *Human energy requirements: a manual for planners and nutritionists.* Oxford, Oxford Medical Publications, 1990 (published on behalf of the Food and Agriculture Organization of the United Nations).
8. *A comparative study of food consumption data from food balance sheets and household surveys.* Rome, Food and Agriculture Organization of the United Nations, 1983 (FAO Economic and Social Development Paper No. 34).
9. WHO Technical Report Series, No. 477, 1971 (Eighth report of the Joint FAO/WHO Expert Committee on Nutrition).
10. FAO Food and Nutrition Series, No. 23, 1988 (*Requirements of vitamin A, iron, folate and vitamin B_{12}*: report of a Joint FAO/WHO Expert Consultation).
11. NATIONAL RESEARCH COUNCIL. *Nutrient adequacy: assessment using food consumption surveys.* Washington, DC, National Academy Press, 1986.
12. LIFE SCIENCES RESEARCH OFFICE. *Guidelines for the use of dietary intake data.* Bethesda, MD, Federation of American Societies for Experimental Biology, 1986.
13. WHO Technical Report Series, No. 452, 1970 (*Requirements of ascorbic acid, vitamin D, vitamin B_{12}, folate and iron*: report of a Joint FAO/WHO Expert Group).
14. BEATON, G.H. & SWISS, L.D. Evaluation of the nutritional quality of food supplies: prediction of "desirable" or "safe" protein:calorie ratios. *American journal of clinical nutrition,* **27**: 485–504 (1974).

A NUTRITIONAL APPROACH TO FOOD LABELLING

The Codex Alimentarius Commission used to suggest that the public needed only to know about the energy, protein, total carbohydrate, and total fat content of a food to gain an adequate view of its nutritional content. However, such an approach can no longer be considered adequate since the content of saturated fatty acids, free sugars, salt, and fibre is also very important from a health point of view. In some developed countries, consumers are already demanding that such information be made available and therefore the Codex proposal for labelling what is known as the "big four" no longer meets the consumer's wishes or needs. Methods therefore need to be devised to help the consumer comprehend additional information.

Some manufacturers, retailers, and caterers have now started to provide information, but consumer surveys show that, in addition to numerical information about nutrients, the public wants a simple "at a glance" method of recognizing the nutrient content of foods. In an effort to aid public understanding, retailers, caterers, local education authorities, and health education officers in some countries have already begun to use systems that divide foods into nutrient categories of high, medium, and low. This shows both the importance attached to simple messages and the desire for some overt expression of the nutrient content of the food. At present the systems vary both in the way they define the different nutrient categories, and in the way in which claims are made. All of the existing systems of grouping into categories have also been determined on subjective grounds, with little or no reference to scientific or medical information.

This variety of approaches to labelling and to categorizing is undesirable from the public's point of view, and the public has a right to be protected from a multiplicity of unspecified methods. It is also undesirable from the food industry's point of view, since the industry, in endeavouring to respond to public demand, is open to criticisms of self-interest in its choice of category limits and the selective way in which it may use labelling.

This issue should be addressed by the Codex Alimentarius Commission and by governments who wish to deal with it as part of their regulations on food labelling. Nevertheless, the present report provides one possible basis for categorizing nutrient contents on food labels, since population nutrient goals have now been established for each of the important dietary components. This may help in rationalizing the present confusion, caused by a range of arbitrary cut-off points for specifying the nutrient content of a food as high, medium, or low.

Before the proposals are set out, however, two issues need to be considered: the applicability of these proposals to developing countries and the appropriateness of specifying the nutrient content of each food in terms of a goal, when it is the overall diet that is important. The use of a population goal for individual purposes might also seem at variance with the theme of this report.

Food labelling in developing countries

It is impossible to label fresh foods sold in local or central markets and the issue of food labelling only really applies to food processed by manufacturers, who sell it in packages or tins that usually have printed labels specifying its nature.

Many countries have a very limited range of food manufacturers and these firms are often very small. To impose on them the burden of specifying the nutrient content of their foods could thus be seen to be unreasonable. Nevertheless, many countries are seeing a rapid development of their food industries and approaches could be devised for helping consumers without imposing great costs on the manufacturer. In the following sections it is suggested that both numerical and simple graphic displays are needed on the labels. The first deals with the actual nutrient content of the food specified in factual terms, e.g., grams of nutrient per 100 g. This gives the impression of considerable accuracy and therefore presupposes the need for detailed reliable and repeated analyses. In practice, considerable progress has been made in establishing the nutrient content of indigenous foods in developing countries, so a nutritionist in the ministry of agriculture could probably advise on the typical nutrient content of a number of foods used in food processing and this could then be presented on the packet as a "typical nutrient content", considerable latitude in the composition of the food being allowed if governments wish to establish food standards.

A much simpler scheme would involve only a graphic display. This method could simply have three categories for each of the nutrients of concern and each category would cover an appreciable range of nutrient compositions. It would therefore allow some latitude for variation in food manufacturing practices and would also not demand of the consumer an understanding of how to integrate all the dietary items in a weekly menu, or of how to convert a figure for nutrients in grams per 100 g into a meaningful term in relation to his or her food needs.

Thus it might be seen as reasonable to introduce graphic labelling first in developing countries using a visual display appropriate to the country. Clearly, in each country the types of food, stage of development, culture, and technical resources differ, but as the expansion of urban communities accelerates the need for food preservation, packaging, and processing is likely to increase, making it more difficult for the population to respond effectively to nutrition and health education without some form of information on food products.

Labelling and categorizing of individual foods

This report emphasizes the importance of community involvement in both the policy-making and the policy-implementation stages of a country's programme for encouraging food patterns appropriate for health. Information for consumers is therefore important, but the challenge is one of educating consumers so that they can exercise their free choice when purchasing foods, on the basis of a knowledge of the content of the foods and how dietary patterns affect health. Some would claim that allowing people to make a free choice in the full knowledge of what they are doing is almost impossible. In developed countries consumers often go to supermarkets with tens of thousands of different food items on display. The informed consumer wishing to choose a healthy diet must then cope with interpreting the food labels while recognizing that it is the overall diet that is important and not the individual food items. Experts often emphasize the importance of achieving a variety and balance of food items to ensure nutritional adequacy and that no foods should be characterized as "good" or "bad". On this basis, the consumer is now provided in many developed countries with most packaged food items displaying an extensive list of nutrients expressed on a weight basis i.e., x mg per 100 g of food. It is still unclear whether consumers attempt to integrate all this information and relate it to the different energy needs of their families, with perhaps a threefold variation in energy requirements between individuals within the family. This is an area to which health educators, consumer organizations, and food manufacturers have not given enough attention.

The following sets of proposals are developed as a first attempt to cope with these problems. It should be recognized that the proposals stem from nutritional and health principles, whereas the present methods of display depend mainly on the traditional approaches of food chemists, food technologists, and legislators. The present proposals may be considered more useful to consumer needs.

Nutrients expressed in relation to food energy

Table 13 of the main report (page 108) expressed all the nutritional goals initially in terms of total energy content except for dietary cholesterol, dietary fibre, and salt, which were originally studied for their effects in relation to their actual intakes expressed on a weight basis. There is, however, no evidence that the weight of the food normally determines the amount consumed, because it is increasingly evident that when food is freely available, appetite control based on energy needs is surprisingly precise in humans. With very bulky diets in selected developing countries, mothers and young children may not be able to eat enough to satisfy their energy requirements. Bulky foods may, as noted in section 3, also help to limit energy intakes in adults, but the overall effect is small and may amount to only a small proportion of the total energy ingested. Children and adults normally eat to meet their energy needs, the amount of food eaten being adjusted subconsciously over a period of days so that it approximates the individual's rate of energy expenditure. This adjustment in appetite and food intake is under powerful physiological control and occurs despite the different water and energy contents of foods.

On this basis, it is simple to specify that in practice the primary demand is for food energy, but very few people have any knowledge or understanding of what their energy needs are. Individual energy needs vary substantially, depending on constitutional (probably genetic) factors, size, age, sex, and the amount of physical activity taken. It is therefore not easy even for an expert to predict an individual's energy requirement and there may be a 20% error in the prediction amounting in an adult man to an error of up to 5 MJ per day (1200 kcal$_{th}$). Intrinsic personal control of energy intake is much more accurate than this, so it could be argued that specifying food energy is of little importance for consumers unless they wish simply to see that the food contains some, a little, or a great deal of energy, or if they wish to attempt to work out over a matter of weeks their energy needs by laboriously measuring the food's energy content and monitoring their own body weight. This approach is clearly irrelevant to any community-based health promotion programme which has the objective of maintaining health within a community with diverse energy needs. This report is concerned with the nutritional quality of the diet once a population (or individual) has satisfied its energy requirements, and it is to this issue of nutritional quality rather than energy content that food labelling should be addressed.

With these arguments in mind, it would seem best to include the energy content of foods on the label, but perhaps to express the other nutrients in terms of the energy content of the food. By this means, individuals will be able to learn in a more meaningful way about the nutrient density of foods and therefore integrate more simply the numerous items in their diet. Even this is difficult, however, since with numerical labelling there is still a requirement for mathematical skills; this approach makes an unreasonable demand on most consumers. Concern for a simpler scheme has led to the following suggestions for labels that indicate grouping into categories on a nutritional basis. If grouping on a numerical basis in terms of energy units is unacceptable because of the need to refer to the weight of the food, then the following grouping systems might need to be expressed symbolically in terms of energy. The symbols will identify whether the nutrient content is in the high, medium or low category, but there is no intrinsic reason for the basis of the symbols to be displayed.

Categorizing the nutrient content of foods

It seems reasonable to expect that consumers will have only a crude understanding of their nutrient needs, but their understanding might be helped if there were some simple scheme for categorizing the nutrient content of foods. This has led some retailers with extensive supermarket chains in developed countries to label their foods as having a high, medium or low content of a particular nutrient.

This report specifies upper and lower limits for the population's average nutrient intake of a number of nutrients, which have not, until recently, been specified on food labels. If public health policy is to succeed through consumer information and education, then it may be useful to have some consistency in approach. For example, nutrient goals specified in this report could be used to specify category ranges. Table A6.1 shows the proposed categories and the items that it might be reasonable to label. Where no lower population limit figure is given, it is suggested that the lower limit should be 50% of the upper limit, which in all cases corresponds to the population average. It is probably not necessary to label and categorize all the items given in Table A6.1, but discussions on how much to include might well be undertaken by a board for nutrition and food policy.

Table A6.1. Summary of a possible approach to the indication of nutrient content categories on food labels for the purpose of consumer education [a]

Nutrient	Low	Medium	High
* Total fat (% energy)	<15	15–30	>30
* Saturated fatty acids (% energy)	<5	5–10	>10
Polyunsaturated fatty acids (% energy)	<3	3–7	>7
Dietary cholesterol (mg/10 MJ energy)	<150	150–300	>300
Total carbohydrate (% energy)	<55	55–75	>75
Complex carbohydrate (% energy)	<50	50–70	>70
Total dietary fibre (g/10 MJ energy)	<27	27–40	>40
* Non-starch polysaccharides (g/10 MJ energy)	<16	16–24	>24
* Free sugars (% energy)	<5	5–10	>10
* Salt (g/10 MJ energy)	<3	3–6	>6

[a] The units are all expressed in terms of energy but it is expected that these numbers will not appear on labels—simply some graphic representation of "high", "medium", or "low".

The total dietary fibre values are approximately equivalent to the sum of the values obtained by the new method of analysis for both non-starch polysaccharides and resistant starch. Current values in European food tables depend substantially on an enzymic method, which gives values that include both non-starch polysaccharides and resistant starch. The resistant starch content of foods is variable and can readily be manipulated by manufacturing and other techniques.

Although the total content of sugars may be used in providing the numerical information on a food's composition, it would be more helpful, from an educational point of view, for the category system to indicate free sugars instead. For simplicity, only the nutrients marked with an asterisk should be included in a graphic display. Non-starch polysaccharides may be separated from other nutrients on the label, since they are the only food components for which a high content is considered beneficial. Although the protein content of a food may be included in numerical labelling for legal purposes, its inclusion in a simplified graphic display for consumers is less necessary.

In Annex 5, it is shown that an individual goal may be specified at a different level from the population average. Thus, an individual may be advised that a total fat intake below 30% of energy would be preferable and values of 20% have been suggested. In this report, no attempt has been made to set individual goals, so it seems appropriate to take the population goal for the purposes of food labelling. Consumers will then only have to balance the number of food items in the low, medium, and high categories to achieve a diet which, with suitable recognition of the dominance of certain food items in the diet, will emerge as having a nutrient content between the lower and upper population limits. This assumes that the amount of energy of the different food items has been taken into account to some extent, but it does simplify the process of decision-making by consumers, as illustrated in the following tabulation:

Standard route for integrating information from food labels	Use of nutrient categories, expressed on an energy basis
1. Add all nutrient weights individually for each food over a day or a week 2. Estimate own energy requirements (only possible in very approximate terms) 3. Convert nutrient intake to energy 4. Calculate nutrient intakes as proportions of energy ingested.	1. Balance high, medium, and low items 2. Not necessary to estimate own energy requirements 3. Ensure that energy obtained from high and low nutrient categories is approximately the same, and that foods in the medium nutrient category are an important part of the diet.

WORLD HEALTH ORGANIZATION
TECHNICAL REPORT SERIES

Recent reports:

* Prices in developing countries are 70% of those listed here.